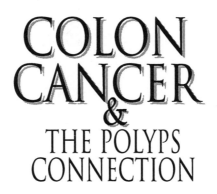

COLON CANCER
&
THE POLYPS
CONNECTION

Stephen Fisher

Illustrated
by David Fischer

FISHER
er
BOOKS™

Publishers: Bill Fisher
Helen Fisher
Howard Fisher

Editors: Sarah Smith
Scott Millard

Book Production: Deanie Wood

Art Director: B. Josh Young

Illustrations: David Fischer

Published by Fisher Books
4239 West Ina Road, Suite 101
Tucson, Arizona 85741
(520) 744-6110

**Library of Congress
Cataloging-in-Publication Data**

Fisher, Stephen J., 1943-
    Colon cancer & the polyps
    connection/Stephen Fisher;
    illustrated by David Fischer.
        p.   cm.
    Includes bibliographical
    references and index.
    ISBN 1-55561-080-3
    1. Colon (Anatomy)—Cancer.
    2. Intestinal polyps.
    I. Title.
RC280.C6F57 1995
616.99' 4347—dc20   95-17803
                                  CIP

Notice: The information in this book is true and complete to the best of our knowledge. It is offered with no guarantees on the part of the author or Fisher Books. Author and publisher disclaim all liability in connection with the use of this book.

Dedication

to Nanci . . . and tomorrow

I am enthralled and at ease,
not for today
but for tomorrow.
Today's moment I take for granted.
Tomorrow will last forever.

Table of Contents

Section II Prevention: The Impact of Diet

Appendixes

Foreword

BY DR. HENRY F. SAFRIT

Today's physicians seek their inspiration from many different sources. I was greatly inspired by a recent visit to the famous Ether Dome at Massachusetts General Hospital in Boston. On October 16, 1846, this wonderful, historic surgical amphitheater was the site of the first public demonstration of ether as an effective anesthesia in surgical operations. The surgeon was John C. Warren. The anesthesia was administered by a dentist, Dr. William T. G. Morton. Robert Hinckley captured the drama of the occasion in a beautiful painting that hangs in the Francis A. Countway Library of Medicine, Boston Medical Library in Cambridge.

This event, along with so many other great discoveries of the 19th century, ushered in the age of modern medicine. The pace of discovery is ever-quickening. In the past 50 years we've witnessed:

- Effective prevention of many infectious diseases (such as polio and diphtheria) by immunization.
- Cure of many infectious diseases with antibiotics.
- Cure of many cancers with refined surgical procedures, radiation and chemotherapy.
- Prolongation of life in patients with cardiovascular disease by recognizing the value of diet as therapy, the use of drugs, and with angioplasty and surgery.

Today's technology has introduced such dramatic "tools" as arthroscopy, fiberoptic flexible colonoscopy, bronchoscopy and laser.

Another important phenomenon which occurred in medicine in more recent years is the increasing involvement of patients in the decision-making process of medical care. In ever-greater numbers, patients want to know more about their diseases and more about the treatments available to them. As a result, there is a growing medical literature written for the non-professional.

This leads me to another source of recent inspiration. Most often, literature for the patient population is written by the medical profession. As curious as patients have become, still few medical publications have come from this lay population. Researching and writing by the non-professional on medical subjects is no easy task. Yet, here we have a patient,

Stephen Fisher, who discovered a colonic polyp and, even after his successful treatment, wanted to know more about his disease. He was not satisfied with the published information so he researched and wrote a book of his own on the subject.

Though colon cancer and its relationship with colonic polyps is far from being perfectly understood, careful study and accumulated data suggest a more aggressive approach to the treatment of colon polyps is appropriate, with resulting successful outcome and cure. This point of view is reflected in Mr. Fisher's carefully organized book. The book is full of factual information and sound conclusions. It is easy to read and will be valuable to anyone who has colorectal cancer or polyps—or who has an interest in the subject. The author's efforts represent the ultimate involvement in one's disease. This book is another positive example of how far we have come in our efforts to advance medical care since that historic day in the Ether Dome in 1846.

HENRY F. SAFRIT, M.D.
    Chief, Division of Endocrinology
        California Pacific Medical Center
    Clinical Professor of Medicine
        University of California
        San Francisco, California

Foreword

BY DR. ROBERT D. TUFFT

This book will save many lives, possibly yours or that of a loved one.

It was written to help the layperson understand and prevent colorectal cancer. It is an excellent resource for everyone and thoroughly explains the complex subjects of colon-cancer screening and the diseases of colonic polyps and colon carcinoma. At some time in their lives, five to six percent of all people in the United States will develop colorectal cancer. Colorectal cancer accounts for 15 percent of all newly diagnosed cancers and is the second most frequent cause of cancer deaths in the United States.

Few people realize that colorectal cancer is preventable and can be easily screened. Most people are aware of the importance of cancer screening and the importance of mammography and pap tests. Yet few realize the importance and equal necessity of colon-cancer screening and the tests involved in such screening. Not many people realize that colon-cancer risk can be reduced by dietary modifications, just as lung-cancer risks can be reduced by stopping smoking.

In 1980, the American Cancer Society recommended screening sigmoidoscopies for Americans at age 50 and then every three to five years thereafter. Although these were the recommendations, only one-fifth of Americans have had any screening sigmoidoscopies. The medical profession and the patient should be more aggressive in following the Cancer Society's screening recommendations.

In today's complex society with its complex health-care system, one must, as a patient, regularly take an active role to ensure that one's care is proper. The author, Mr. Fisher, arms the readers of this book with all the information they need to become informed health-care consumers and to protect their own health. He guides the reader to proper care in cancer prevention, whether the reader is a healthy person or one afflicted with colorectal cancer.

Diseases such as cancer are thieves that rob us of our health, steal our happiness and weaken our spirit. As frail human beings, knowledge is our best weapon against disease. This book imparts the knowledge necessary to fight for health and, as previously stated, will save many readers' lives.

ROBERT D. TUFFT, M.D.
   Diplomate, American Board
      of Internal Medicine
   Summit Hospital, Oakland, California

Prologue
Discovery and Reactions

My annual physical examination results came back well within acceptable guidelines. In fact, for a 50-year-old man, cholesterol and blood pressure were impressively on the low side. But, during the rectal exam, Dr. Taylor discovered a slight trace of blood. While giving assurances that it was nothing serious, he made arrangements for me to get a more in-depth examination from a specialist.

Several weeks later, I finally found time to visit Dr. Sada. During the first appointment, he preformed a procedure which he called a *sigmoidoscopy*. At the time, it was as if he was speaking Greek. I could not even pronounce the word. And I could not understand why I next had to go to the hospital to have a *colonoscopy*. But, he was the doctor. Although I didn't like the idea of interrupting my busy schedule, I decided that following the expert's advice would be the intelligent course of action.

I had the colonoscopy the following week, and quickly forgot about Dr. Sada and his outrageous tests—until the morning of October 30, 1992. The telephone call from Dr. Sada was totally unexpected. It was a call that changed my life forever.

"The test results came back positive," he said in a matter-of-fact voice. "You have the beginning of cancer on the tip of a polyp."

The doctor's call put me on an emotional roller coaster as I attempted to deal with an abrupt awakening to a new set of life's priorities, accompanied by fears I had never before experienced.

Writing has always been an outlet for me. Without any forethought, the startling news triggered the beginning of a personal journal that I kept from the moment I was first advised of my cancer until the final treatment. The material in this section is a condensed version of the diary, tracing my crusade to discover the source of my problem and to identify the ramifications.

All of the doctors' names have been changed.

Day 1—October 30th (Friday)

Is having the "beginning of cancer" the same as being "a little bit pregnant"? The idea that it always happens to somebody else—accompanied by my unconscious beliefs of invincibility—were quickly destroyed by Dr. Sada's report over the telephone. It is odd how that word "cancer" stays with me. And, I wonder, what is a polyp? Isn't it a flower?

I'm not sure what I am supposed to do or how I'm supposed to feel. Where there is a beginning, there is an end.

I guess, in my narrow perspective, the end of cancer is death. I wonder, am I going to die? Suddenly, two thoughts begin to bother me. My first thought is that I feel great. If I have the "beginning of cancer," you would think that I should be sick. My second thought is that I am not afraid of dying. But curiously, up until an hour ago, I never before even thought about *me* dying.

I wonder how it will end. My mind is muddled and rushing with all kinds of thoughts, none of them pleasant. How will I react to pain? . . . maybe I should retire . . . am I overreacting? Well, keep cool! I know how to handle this thing! I'm going to go home, open a bottle of good wine and get smashed.

Day 2—October 31st (Saturday)

I slept a solid six hours last night, I suppose due to the effects of the wine. But, I woke up startled this morning, with my eyes wide open and one thought in my mind: *I have cancer.*

I have decided that I am not going to change my life. I am going to maintain my business routine as if nothing is wrong. Then, I am going to attack this cancer thing with an organized, sensible approach. Beginning on Monday, I'll initiate Phase One of my Cancer Strategic Plan: I'll find another doctor to get a second opinion. I'll also learn what "beginning of cancer" actually means. And I'm going to start a new diet.

I am not comfortable with Dr. Sada. I have the feeling he puts himself together every day by inserting himself into a "doctor" mold. After all is said and done, this guy sticks a pole up my butt, finds something called a *polyp*, cuts off the head and somehow leaves the stalk. He jolts me with an abrupt telephone call, coldly advising me I have cancer. Now, next week, he wants me to go back into the hospital so that he can have a second chance at getting out the stalk. My "Dr. Sada" experience is not formulated around the elements of confidence. Well, I'd better move on quickly.

But my mind is running like a locomotive with this cancer thing. I think it is the newness . . . it must be the newness. I wonder how I will react when I settle down into routine day-to-day coping with this problem. My thought process now seems confused and crystal-clear at the same time.

Day 3—November 1st (Sunday)

Last night was the first time I had socialized since being told I had cancer. During the evening, the thought of cancer was never far away from me. As the night progressed, there seemed to be a detachment where I heard people talking, but I could not hear the words. During 20 years of marriage, I have never hidden anything from Nanci. I am dreading the idea of telling her.

Today, we watched the New York Marathon from our living-room windows, then went out to the street to get closer to the action. While standing on the sidewalk with the crowd, I just started crying. Thank God I was wearing my dark glasses. Obviously, I have something going on in the depths of my soul that is different from anything I've ever experienced before.

Nanci and I are completely entwined. When one hurts, laughs or cries, the other feels the same emotion. It's as if we have grown and matured as individuals, sharing a common emotional core. She keeps asking me what is wrong. I will tell her tomorrow.

Day 4—November 2nd (Monday)

It has been five years since I last spoke to Dr. Miller in Pittsburgh, but it was like catching up with an old friend. After I had explained my situation, he advised me to call Dr. Jones in New York.

Good-bye Dr. Miller in Pittsburgh; hello Dr. Jones in New York City. After two hours of confronting a busy telephone at Dr. Jones' office, frustration got the best of me. I took a cab down the yellow brick road into the mysterious, scary world of pretentious New York City medicine. Constantly busy telephones and a near-5th Avenue office address should have served as a warning.

Walking into Dr. Jones' office was like walking into a New York horse-race betting parlor. Three women in the reception room were handling a constant stream of incoming telephone calls. I approached the desk closest to the office door. Receptionist #1 looked up at me with a glare that was apparently intended to scare me away. I decided I must look like a salesman. Finally, in desperation (or exasperation), Receptionist #1 put the caller on hold and asked me what I wanted. Her voice was loud enough to alert everyone in the office.

"Dr. Miller at Allegheny General recommended that I see Dr. Jones," I replied.

"Dr. Jones is not taking any new patients."

"Why don't you just tell Dr. Jones . . ."

"What's your problem?"

"I have been diagnosed as having cancer."

As difficult as it was for me to say those words, I knew that they would not sound earth-shattering to her. But I was not prepared for her bored "What's the big deal?" look and immediate dismissal.

"We don't have the time . . ."

"Lady, are you trying to put me on the defensive?"

Finally realizing that I was not going to budge until she took some sort of action, she wrote down details of my medical history. New York is undoubtedly a tough place. It will be interesting to see if the doctor calls me tomorrow, as Receptionist #1 promised.

The day is over and I am not sure if I accomplished anything. Now, I am just trying to keep my cool.

The lead story in today's *New York Times* sports section was about Jim Valvano's experiences with cancer and his upcoming return to broadcasting. He relates that his greatest life experience was not the upset winning of the national collegiate basketball championship. Rather, it was the people he met during the fight to regain his life after being diagnosed with cancer.

Yesterday, the wheelchair marathoners and marathon founder Fred LeBow (with his brain cancer in remission) exhibited their dedication to survival and achievement, regardless of the odds. Funny how quickly one finds new heroes.

Day 5—November 3rd (Tuesday)

In all honesty, I really did not care if Dr. Jones called. But the persistent shoot-from-the-hip, decision-oriented approach to business that I have nurtured over the years forced me to go back to his office. In retrospect, I guess that curiosity was also a motivating factor.

Again, I entered the office and walked over to Receptionist #1. She looked up in disbelief.

This time she was more quick to put her caller on hold. She spoke in the voice that a teacher uses when scolding a child. "What are *you* doing here?"

"I'm sick."

"This is a doctor's office."

"I thought doctors' offices were good places for sick people to go."

"It is inappropriate for you to come into this office. Dr. Jones is too busy to take new patients—with or without cancer."

What else could I say? New York is just a tough place. Forget it! Move on!

I only hope that I can keep this thing from becoming a "big deal." Thousands of people get cancer every day. It is a mental game that I have to keep in perspective. I must react fast and decisively. I think my greatest danger is feeling sorry for myself.

I'm not sure what is worse—having cancer or not telling Nanci the truth. I find I am always looking for that perfect time to break the bad news. But when an opportunity presents itself, I unconsciously invent some excuse that allows me to postpone the inevitable. On one hand, I'm plagued with guilt because of my cover-up. On the other hand, I compliment myself for protecting her another day. Sometime, somewhere, I have to come to grips with this miserable situation and tell Nanci what's going on. I am just a coward.

Day 6—November 4th (Wednesday)

Dr. Jones' office called today. It was none other than Receptionist #1 on the line. She informed me: "Dr. Jones will not be seeing you. Dr. Baker will see you on Monday at 1:00 p.m. You must bring with you all records, slides and films. There will be a $350 consultation fee that must be paid on Monday."

I wonder if I have to pay the $350 before seeing the doctor.

Yes, this has to be New York. Just think—if these are "teaching doctors" responsible for molding a new generation of medical professionals, we are going to have monsters.

I canceled Dr. Baker's appointment. Surely, I'm not interested in any doctor who feels as if he's doing me a special favor.

I still do not have a doctor.

All day yesterday I had been rehearsing and scheming how to tell Nanci. Only in New York can you go to a different good restaurant every night of the year. Yet, we usually end up in one of a few nearby restaurants where everybody is on a first-name basis. My carefully conceived plans included dinner at our quiet corner table at McMullins.

I had let everything build up so much inside me, my guts were squirming. I was sure that the anxiety was showing on my face when we met at the restaurant. On cue, after the waiter left the bottle of wine at the table, I was ready to launch into my speech. But I simply forgot all my carefully rehearsed words as I blurted out, "I have something to tell you—don't worry or overreact."

I could see the tears welling up in her eyes and her lips began to quiver. For a split second, I tried to figure out what else I could say to change the subject and escape once again. But it was too late. After the passage of a few quiet seconds, I conjured up all my savvy and eloquence and said, simply: "I have been diagnosed with colon cancer." The anguish in her face would not go away. We barely sipped the wine and left without dinner. While a giant weight had been lifted from my shoulders, I really didn't feel any better as we walked home together, quiet, tightly holding hands.

Day 7—November 5th (Thursday)

After a sleepless night, Nanci was back in control yesterday morning with nonstop questions. She certainly recaptured *her* composure. She is ready for the doctors. I doubt the doctors will be ready for her!

My pants seem to fit a little looser today. Maybe I've reached the stage where I'm losing weight. Instead of my usual bowl of cereal, I ate seven jelly donuts for breakfast.

I called old, dependable Dr. Joe Grant in San Francisco this morning. He wasted no time in getting to the heart of the matter. "Call Fred Carter at Sloan-Kettering and tell him you are a friend of mine." Apparently, Dr. Carter is not the doctor for me. But I am hopeful he will direct me to the right person.

Will wonders ever cease? I have found a real doctor in New York! After a brief introduction on the telephone, Dr. Carter responded quickly. "You should see Dr. Brown at Sloan-Kettering. What day is best for you? I will make arrangements and call you at your office to confirm."

Day 8—November 6th (Friday)

I was wrong about losing weight. I forgot that of my six pairs of gray slacks, one has a slightly larger waist than the others. And that was the pair I wore yesterday. In addition to the seven jelly donuts I had for breakfast, I ate four peanut-butter cups, a large bag of potato chips, a couple of candy bars, two hamburgers with a large order of fries plus a giant sausage hero!

Not surprisingly, I could barely button my regular-size slacks this morning. And my belt had to be extended to the next notch.

I keep studying myself in the mirror, expecting changes . . . but I do not see any difference in the way I look.

Day 9—November 7th (Saturday)

At last, my focus can now shift from finding a doctor to gaining a true understanding of the problem. I want to learn the ramifications and my options. It's certain I cannot allow my current mind-set to continue. I will probably go crazy if my thoughts constantly wander back to that cancer word.

I am anxiously awaiting Tuesday morning's appointment with Dr. Brown. I hope I can gain some better insight into this thing. I feel confident Dr. Brown will be the right doctor for me. For sure, Sloan-Kettering is the right place to be. It is a good place to "play the game" when the "arena" is located almost next door.

I have already started preparing my agenda of questions for the doctor:

•What books should I read?
•What should be my diet?
•What are the immediate and long-term dangers
    and ramifications?
•What is the worst-case scenario confronting me?

Day 11—November 9th (Monday)

Tonight, for the first time, I feel really depressed. Maybe I am feeling sorry for myself. Whatever it is, this low feeling is reaching down to the pit of my stomach. I'm not sure how to react. I think the hardest part of coping with this thing is that from the beginning I've had a feeling of losing control. Funny, I have tears in my eyes. I guess I am just tired.

Day 12—November 10th (Tuesday)

Where do I start? It has been less than two weeks since the news, but it seems more like two years that this ominous cloud has been hanging over my head.

The single word that best sums up my first impression of Sloan-Kettering is "civility." It is open, warm and clean. Most important, the people are courteous and caring.

In fact, in my experience, Sloan-Kettering seems unique. I find it difficult to understand why anyone in the medical profession is not first endowed with humanity and humility. Sloan-Kettering is synonymous with cancer. There is a feeling of pleasant efficiency to the place. It provides confidence to the person who walks through the front door, most of whom are scared and bewildered. There is an unspoken attitude here that says: "If you've got cancer, this is the place to be."

Dr. Brown is a surgeon and a leading authority on cancer in the digestive areas of the body. He makes a typical doctor's first impression . . . mid-60s, a little heavyset and bald. He seems to be a very efficient person with a dry sense of humor who is also capable of making fun of himself.

I do not think that Dr. Brown was very impressed with the slide and report from Dr. Sada. In his office, he studied the slide under a microscope. His conclusion was that it was important for me to have another colonoscopy. Not bad! I can write and pronounce the word now. It is amazing how medical terminology so quickly becomes part of your everyday vocabulary when confronting a serious illness.

Dr. Brown's secretary has scheduled the dreaded colonoscopy procedure for this coming Friday. It will be performed by Dr. Jim Johnson who, you could say, is the "head colonoscopy man" at Sloan-Kettering.

Ironic. For 50 years, no medical person touched me. Now, within a period of 19 days, I'll have had a sigmoidoscopy and two colonoscopies.

If you have any pride or dignity, it quickly evaporates with a rectal illness. Dr. Brown's recommendation that I have a colonoscopy led to a flashback of my visit to Roosevelt Hospital just a couple of weeks ago. It was then that Dr. Sada and his cohorts (I labeled them by their job duties: a cleaner, a holder and a pusher) worked on my bare butt as I lay helpless on a tabletop in a small, sterile, nondescript room. How does it feel? I honestly can't explain how having strangers pushing a pipe up your butt feels. You just grit your teeth and get through it. Strangely, I wonder if all these doctors and nurses ever experience any morale problems as they head off "to the office" for another day of this type of work?

If the colonoscopy itself wasn't bad enough, the body-cleansing preparations that are required the night before are infinitely worse. It begins with a prescription for a gallon jug that looks like the plastic bottles of spring water you buy at the supermarket. The jug is empty of liquid, but at the bottom is a mysterious powdered material. The instructions tell you to fill the bottle with water and shake to mix the powder. Starting at 6:00 p.m. the night before the colonoscopy, you are instructed to drink a glass of this foul-tasting liquid—*every 10 minutes!* After about three hours, it hits you like a bomb. Until you experience it, you never knew a human body could hold so much. You get up from the toilet to have another drink, which you finish only in time to run back to the toilet.

But, this isn't the whole preparation procedure. The doctor's printed instructions call for an enema before you go to sleep and one when you get up. Before buying the first Fleet® enemas, I had never even thought about enemas, much less had one!

At about 11:00 p.m., when I thought that there could not possibly be anything left in me, I read the package instructions and studied the diagrams on the enema box. Sprawled out naked on the living-room floor, I did my best to follow the instructions. I put my body through a series of never-before-attempted contortions and experimented with about a half-dozen positions. Finally, after the frustration that always accompanies multiple failures of trying anything new, I was successful.

Early the next morning, before leaving for that first colonoscopy appointment, I repeated the enema process. This time it was easy. I guess it's like riding a bicycle. Once you learn, you never forget.

Considering that the Roosevelt Hospital colonoscopy done by Dr. Sada was not entirely successful—I still had the polyp stalk inside me—I agreed with Dr. Brown that I should have a second colonoscopy. So here we go again. Thank God it's Friday: time for another colonoscopy!

Oh yes. Having "the beginning of cancer" is not like being "a little bit pregnant." As Dr. Brown explained: "Having cancer is like a tiger in a cage. It is dangerous but controllable. In your case, the tiger is merely sticking his nose out of the bars."

I am not sure I completely understand Dr. Brown's explanation. To be truthful, he did not make me feel any better. He did say that I should start thinking about a high-fiber diet, but he wanted to see the results of the colonoscopy before making any definite recommendations.

Day 13—November 11th (Wednesday)

The remarkable feature of my consciousness is that physically I feel wonderful . . . but, mentally, I know only sickness. My consciousness is constantly haunted with thoughts of the cancer inside me.

Day 15—Friday the 13th

Can you believe it? It is Friday the 13th and I am on my way to Sloan-Kettering for *Colonoscopy Number Two!*

Day 16—November 14th (Saturday)

Yesterday, after an excellent, relaxing dinner at the Museum Cafe, we picked up a videocassette on the way home. As soon as we climbed into bed, turned out the lights and put on the movie, I started crying—again. This is getting out of hand!

I lay in bed trying to understand this new crying habit. I don't feel scared. I am no longer even worried. As soon as I placed myself into Sloan-Kettering and under Dr. Brown's care, I rationalized that under the circumstances everything has been done that could be done. At the risk of being trite, I now have to "keep my head up," "roll with the punches" and "play the hand that has been dealt." Constant worrying will not achieve anything. I don't think I'm feeling sorry for myself.

I guess I was tired and relieved at the same time after the colonoscopy. That's understandable. And there *was* that extra added excitement!

The morning began with a series of Sloan-Kettering introductory interviews before I was ushered into the operating room. It was like being beamed down onto the flight deck of the Starship Enterprise in the middle of a *Star Trek* mission. I was in a large room with computers and gleaming medical equipment crammed onto every inch of wall space. The ceiling was filled with hanging lights, tubes and pipes. I was greeted by a half-dozen men and women in green uniforms, ready to work "on the flight deck." This looked to be a well-synchronized team functioning with the efficiency of a rocket-launching crew.

I was told to take off my robe, leaving my loose-fitting, open-backed hospital gown hanging over my shoulders.

Underneath I was naked. I was asked to climb onto a table in the center of the action where I quietly lay on my back as two nurses attached wires to me. They gave detailed explanations as to the purpose of every hook-up, but I was not listening. When they were done, I had a clothespin on one finger and an array of suction-cup electrodes taped to my chest. As the action around me continued, it dawned on me that there had been a mix-up of patients . . . all these busy people were getting me ready for a heart transplant!

After the chief nurse calmed me down and carefully explained everybody's tasks and responsibilities, the copilot, that is, the assisting doctor entered the room. He introduced himself and explained the forthcoming procedure in detail—as if I really needed to hear it all for the second time in a few weeks! He was so intense that I did not have the heart to tell him I was practically a colonoscopy expert.

My colonoscopy was scheduled for 9:00 a.m. and it was already 9:15. I felt compelled to explain to the gathered troops that, in the real business world, people are on time for meetings. "Of course," I said, "I will have to explain to Dr. Johnson the importance of timeliness."

"If someone was going to do to me what Dr. Johnson is going to do to you," replied the nurse, "I would go to great lengths not to say anything to upset him."

Made sense to me. When Dr. Johnson walked into the operating room at about 9:30, I cheerfully asked if he was having a pleasant morning!

"Bottoms up," he said, "and let the work begin."

After my show was over, I was taken to the recovery area. Dr. Johnson came out to explain that they had removed all of the polyp. I should call early next week to get results of the analysis. He then recommended that I join a four-year study group comprised of people who have had polyps removed. The object of the study is to determine whether a bad diet was the cause of polyps and colon cancer. It is called the *PPT*, or *Polyp Prevention Trial.*

After Dr. Johnson left the recovery area, a dietitian came in to explain briefly the polyp study mentioned by Dr. Johnson. I asked her several times about *my* diet, but she politely refused to give me advice. I finally gave up trying to understand the logic of a hospital dietitian refusing to give a patient diet information! Next week, I will call about the polyp study, which, at first glance, appears an excellent way to monitor my condition.

Today, I have settled down. I can for the first time see the light at the end of the tunnel. For all purposes, it's all done for "Phase One." There is nothing else for me to do until I get the results of the colonoscopy next week.

I wonder how it will end.

Day 19—End Game

The colonoscopy was successful, and it is all over for the time being. Dr. Brown said that all the cancer had been removed.

He also stressed that I must always monitor my condition because I am now at high risk of getting more cancer. I'm hopeful I'll be okay. I am undoubtedly a very fortunate person. It's time to get on with life and put everything behind me. Although I'd like to forget about the ordeal, the die has been cast. The experience has made a lasting impression.

Now I know it doesn't always happen to someone else.

About the Author

Steve Fisher is 52 years old. He is the founder and president of Fisher Associates, a computer consulting firm. He is also an author, columnist and lecturer focusing on automated systems and technology applications in business. Professor Fisher was asked to develop and present a special course at Fordham University's School of Business. Steve and his wife, Nanci, have been married for over 20 years. They live in San Francisco and New York.

Section I

Medical Implications

Preface
GETTING PAST THE UNMENTIONABLE WORDS

Certain medical words and terms are taboo in our society. Most people outside the medical profession have difficulty discussing the processes of the digestive system—until they are confronted with a related illness. The American Cancer Society recognizes the natural reluctance of people to focus on the realities of colon cancer and offers this simple piece of advice: "Don't die of embarrassment."

Experience sickness anywhere in your digestive system, and it is amazing how quickly language restraints disappear. There is simply no way to gloss over words that deal with potentially life-threatening medical problems. In fact, discussions about digestive functions should be as open and natural as discussions about heart functions. All parts of the body have particular roles to play in keeping a person healthy and alive.

After years of researching and writing about computers, my sudden confrontation with life-threatening illness launched my investigation into such unfamiliar subjects as *intestines, bowels, anal canal, anus, rectum, excretion, colon*—and *cancer.* My research began as soon as I was exposed to doctors and nurses discussing frightening problems in condescending tones. They used words and terms I did not understand.

My frustration and curiosity forced me into the library. By no means did I intend to become a self-taught medical expert. But people were talking about and doing complex and mysterious things to my body. The medical words were like scattered pieces of a puzzle. Trying to understand the jargon of an impatient doctor was like trying to put a puzzle together without having all the pieces.

This book is not intended to be a sophisticated medical dissertation. Rather, it is written from a patient's point of view in an attempt to provide honest and understandable information on colon cancer. My objective was to become comfortable with my own condition. As my research continued, I discovered it was time well-spent. With the knowledge I gained, I was better equipped to handle problems and questions as they occurred. Ultimately, it allowed me to take an active and intelligent role in the decision-making processes that would affect my health and my life.

About the Notes

Whether it is a book or an article, medical writing in any form is almost always supported by "notes." These notes lead the reader to the authoritative published sources of the writer's comments, claims and conclusions. The same practice has been adopted in Chapters 1 through 9, the medical section of this book. The small numbers appearing in the text correspond to the references listed in the Notes section, pages 223 to 230.

For example, the following statement is made on page 11 in Chapter 2:

There are more than 100 types of cancer.[4]

The list of notes for Chapter 2 begins on page 223, and the published authority for the above statement is given as:

4. NCI, *What You Need to Know About Cancer of the Colon and Rectum* (Publication #90-1552, 1989), 3.

This tells you that the information was found on page 3 of Publication #90-1552, which was produced by the National Cancer Institute in 1989.

1

The Digestive Puzzle
YOUR BODY'S FOOD-PROCESSING SYSTEM

Before beginning a discussion on the subject of colon cancer, it is helpful to have some knowledge concerning the workings of the body's *digestive system*. Also called the *intestinal tract* or the *gastrointestinal tract*, our food-processing system begins at the mouth and ends at the anus. The food we eat travels from the mouth through the *esophagus* (or *gullet*) into the stomach and then into the small intestine (or *small bowel*).[1,2]

The digestive process begins with chewing, the first step in breaking down the food. After food is chewed and swallowed it flows through the esophagus into the stomach, where it is broken down into a loose, fluid form. The stomach regulates the flow into the small bowel, a narrow tube-like organ about 6 meters (20 feet) long. Here the food is converted into substances that can enter the bloodstream and be used throughout the body.[3]

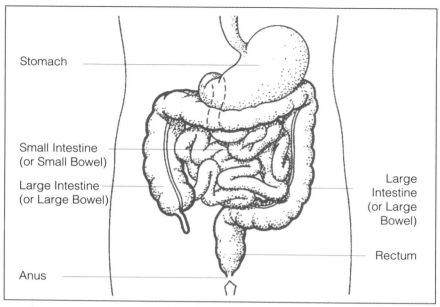

Stomach

Small Intestine
(or Small Bowel)

Large Intestine
(or Large Bowel)

Large
Intestine
(or Large
Bowel)

Rectum

Anus

THE DIGESTIVE SYSTEM

Only 5% to 10% of our food reaches the large bowel, where it is prepared for excretion from the body.[4] The large bowel is much shorter than the small bowel—1.5 to 1.8 meters (five to six feet) in length—but is so named because of its greater diameter, which varies from 2.5 to 7.5cm (one to three inches). It is made up of the *cecum*, the *colon* and the *rectum*.[5]

The colon is shaped like an inverted "U," beginning on the right side and extending upward across the body and down the left side.[6] It is separated into four sections: the *ascending, transverse, descending* and *sigmoid* segments. Its function is to absorb fluids as it processes the remaining food, forming waste material into solids to be excreted.[7]

The last section of the large bowel is the *rectum*. Its primary function is to store food waste (fecal matter or stool) until it is time to excrete it.[8] The *anal canal*, or *anal region*, leads to the body's external opening, the *anus*, through which fecal matter is excreted. The large bowel acts as an efficient assembly line, pushing the stool up, around, down and out of the body.

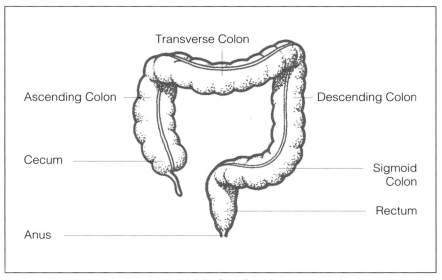

THE LARGE BOWEL

2

Polyps & Bowel Cancer
HIGH RISK & AVERAGE RISK

Cells are the smallest living units of the body capable of independent reproduction, the fundamental building blocks of the body.[1] *Tissues* are collections of similar cells. To repair worn-out or injured cells and to allow for growth, cells normally divide and replace themselves in an orderly, controlled pattern. When this never-ending division of cells becomes disorderly and uncontrolled, too many cells are reproduced and an abnormal growth is formed. The result is a mass of extra tissue known as a *tumor*. A tumor may be *benign*, meaning it is *noncancerous*. Or it may be *malignant*, meaning *cancerous*.[2]

Benign tumors grow in the location where they originated and can possibly interfere with body functions. They are not considered dangerous because they will not spread to other parts of the body, nor will they cause harm to surrounding cells.

The abnormal, uncontrolled growth that we call *cancer* can spread and cause damage throughout the body.[3] There are more than 100 types of cancer.[4] Malignant cells share four important, harmful characteristics:[5]

- A relentless tendency to divide and reproduce.
- A behavior that interferes with the functions of healthy cells.
- A strong inclination to expand and sink roots into surrounding tissues.
- The ability to spread elsewhere in the body.

Polyps

Tumors that grow inside the bowels are called by a variety of names, most often *polyps* or *neoplasms*. You may also hear them referred to as *neoplastic polyps*, *colonic polyps* or *lesions*. Polyps rarely appear in the small bowel, but it is quite common for them to develop in the large bowel.[6] It is estimated that about one-third of the over-50 population in the United States have one or more large-bowel polyps.[7] Every year, over one million people in the U.S. are diagnosed for the first time as having large-bowel polyps.

There are two primary classifications of these polyps. Small *hyperplastic polyps* present little cause for concern.[8] The larger *adenomatous polyps*, often referred to as *adenomas*, are also usually benign but potentially dangerous in that they can evolve into malignancy.[9,10] It is a widely accepted medical premise that most bowel cancers develop from pre-existing adenomas.[11,12] Prompt medical action to remove adenomas is based on the ever-present risk that a newly discovered polyp might be malignant.[13]

However, it is important to point out that only five to ten percent of adenomas become cancerous. Thus, all the bowel cancers might have originated with adenomas, but only a small percentage of the adenomas actually became malignant.[14] When advised that you have an adenoma or an adenomatous polyp, you do not necessarily have cancer. But you are at risk that it will become malignant as the years pass.

The precancerous adenoma usually takes about five years to show signs of malignancy. It is estimated that a benign polyp takes from 5 to 20 years to evolve into "cancer," a process known as the *adenoma-carcinoma sequence*.[15]

The premise that benign adenomas gradually become malignant was documented by a Mayo Clinic study, the results of which were announced in 1987. The study followed the annual examinations of 226 people diagnosed with benign polyps, all of whom elected not to have the polyps removed.[16] From this experience, the researchers concluded that 2.5% of benign polyps will be diagnosed as cancerous after 5 years. In 10 years, the cancer rate will have risen to 8%. After 20 years the cancer-incidence rate reaches 24%.

Polyp Size and Cancer Risk

A polyp may grow to the size of an apple, or larger. As its size increases, so does the risk that the polyp will become malignant.[17] When adenomas grow larger than one centimeter (1cm) in diameter, they are generally considered "large" and have entered a "malignant dangerous zone."[18] In comparison, a cherry is about two centimeters in diameter and a Ping-Pong ball about three centimeters. (1cm = .39 in.)

Large-Bowel Cancer and the Risk Factor

One-third of all people in the Western developed world will get some form of cancer. Cancer causes one-fifth of all reported deaths and is the second-leading cause of all deaths, after heart disease.[19] Figures from the American Cancer Society project that in 1995 there will be about 100,000 new cases of colon cancer and 38,200 new cases of rectal cancer reported in the United States.[20]

Most large-bowel cancer is found in the colon; a smaller percentage develops in the rectum. While different in some respects, both colon and rectum cancer are referred to as *large-bowel cancer, bowel cancer* or *colorectal cancer*. Medical authorities usually employ the term *colorectal cancer*.[21]

High Risk

The designation *high risk* means that a person's chances for getting a disease are greater than those of the general population. It does not mean the person is *destined* to get the disease. While it is impossible to pinpoint with absolute authority the true rate of increased danger, those people at high risk for developing colorectal cancer include:[22, 23, 24, 25]

- Anyone previously diagnosed with bowel cancer or adenomatous polyps.
- Anyone with relatives who have had polyps or bowel cancer, especially if such relatives were under age 55 when these conditions were first detected. The risk is greater for first-degree relationships (parents, siblings or children). The larger the number of relatives with polyps or bowel cancer, the greater the risk.
- Anyone who has had extensive *ulcerative colitis* (numerous ulcers lining the large bowel) for more than 10 years or who suffers from Chron's disease, which is similar. These factors account for about 1% of colorectal-cancer patients.
- Women with a history of breast, ovarian or endometrial cancer.
- Anyone with a parent suffering from *familial polyposis*. In this rare inherited disease, hundreds of polyps develop in the large bowel. *Gardner's syndrome* is a similar condition. About 1% of all cases of colorectal cancer are caused by genetic polyps developing from such diseases.

Average Risk

Everyone who is not in one of the high-risk categories just described is considered to be of *average risk*. There is no *low-risk* category. However, because only 2% to 3% of polyps and colorectal cancer are found in average-risk people under 40 years old, the baseline (or beginning) for average risk is age 40.[26] It is estimated that 55% to 85% of the people who develop colorectal cancer fall into the average-risk category.

Research has provided no clear-cut method for defining the degree of danger for people over 40 years of age.[27] The only point on which all medical authorities agree is that no "safe haven" exists. Every year hundreds of thousands of average-risk people are diagnosed with polyps. And every year tens of thousands of average-risk people are advised that they have colorectal cancer.[28]

Whether you are at average risk or high risk, your position changes with age. After age 50, every passing decade doubles the chances of being diagnosed with adenomas or colorectal cancer. Over 93% of adenomas appear in adults over the age of 50. Various studies indicate that people 65 to 75 years old are in the peak danger period for developing colorectal disorders.[29]

Probability of Developing Colorectal Cancer[30]

Age	0 to 39	40 to 59	60 to 79	Over lifetime
Male	1 in 1667	1 in 110	1 in 22	1 in 16
Female	1 in 2000	1 in 137	1 in 30	1 in 17

Colorectal cancer is the only major cancer that occurs with equal frequency in men and women.[31] The 1995 projections predict that 70,700 men and 67,500 women will be diagnosed with colorectal cancer.[32] Among women, it ranks second after breast cancer. Among men it is the third leading cancer, after prostate cancer and lung cancer. It is estimated that every American has a 1 in 16 chance of developing colorectal cancer in her or his lifetime and that only about half of the newly diagnosed cases will survive for more than five years.[33]

About 3% of all deaths recorded in the United States can be attributed to colorectal cancer.[34] Of all the deaths due to cancer, only lung cancer is more deadly.[35] The predictions for 1995 include 47,500 deaths from colon cancer and 7,800 from rectal cancer.[36]

Both incidence and mortality rates for colorectal cancer have been slowly decreasing during recent years. This small but steady decline is the by-product of improved health awareness, better nutrition, earlier detection, faster diagnosis and advancement in treatment techniques.[37]

3

Polyp Form & the Spread of Cancer

THE PURPOSE OF STAGING

The body's *lymphatic system* is normally the first natural defense mechanism against germs. It produces and stores infection-fighting cells which circulate through the body by means of vessels that resemble blood vessels. Small, rounded, bean-shaped *lymph nodes* are situated at frequent intervals throughout the lymph circulation system. They perform a function similar to that of water-purification plants located on rivers, cleansing the lymph fluid as it passes through. The lymph nodes filter out and destroy waste, bacteria and foreign substances.[1]

Cancer cells can spread throughout the body by means of both the bloodstream and the lymphatic system. Through the bloodstream they reach the body's organs. Through the lymphatic system they go to the nearest lymph nodes. Because the lymph system flows into the blood circulatory system, cancer that has spread into the lymph nodes can also find its way into the bloodstream.[2] Wherever the cancer cells land they can take root and grow. Cells in the new cancer, sometimes called *secondary cancer*, are the same as those found in the original tumor.[3] As this process is repeated, the cancer spreads throughout the body.

The presence of cancer cells in the lymph nodes is an important indication that cancer has spread from its original site.[4] The term *metastasis* is used to identify cancer that has spread. Thus, colon cancer that has spread to the liver is called *colon metastasis* in the liver or *metastasis colon cancer*. For colorectal cancer, metastasis most often takes place in the liver. The second most common area for colon metastasis is the lungs.[5]

Carcinoma is a medical term that describes cancers that arise from the inner lining or surface tissue of an organ such as the large bowel.[6] Carcinomas account for 80% to 90% of all malignant tumors.[7] When a carcinoma is found in the large bowel, there is about a 30% chance of another adenoma and a 2% to 5% chance of another carcinoma being present elsewhere in the large bowel.[8]

Staging

Staging is a method of grading or ranking colorectal cancer. It describes whether the cancer remains within the bowel or has spread to other parts of the body. Staging takes into account how deeply the cancerous tumor has invaded the bowel wall and whether other organs or lymph nodes are involved.[9]

The walls of the digestive tract have four layers of tissue.

The top layer, or *mucosa*, lines the surface of the entire digestive tract from the mouth to the anus. It contains no blood vessels or lymph vessels. Thus, cancer isolated in the mucosa of the large bowel is controllable. The danger of metastasis increases greatly as the cancer penetrates more deeply into the bowel wall where there are blood and lymph vessels that can carry cancer throughout the body.[10]

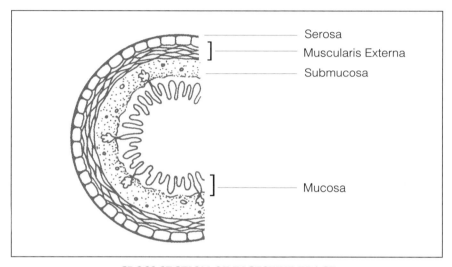

Serosa
Muscularis Externa
Submucosa

Mucosa

CROSS SECTION OF DIGESTIVE TRACT

The first staging method, the *Dukes' System*, was developed in 1932. It ranks and identifies cancer on a scale of A through D. A is least serious. D is most serious.[11]

Since the mid-1980s, the Dukes' System has been refined into the *TNM Staging System*. In this system, T refers to tumor size, N to lymph-node involvement and M to metastasis.[12] The TNM System uses Stage 0 through Stage IV as a standard of measure, with 0 being the least serious and IV being the most serious.

Staging is important because it helps doctors plan the most effective treatment. It also assists them in formulating an intelligent *prognosis* or prediction as to the future course of the illness. For the patient, staging provides insight into the status of his or her current condition. It also offers an opportunity to gain a better understanding of treatment alternatives in the context of how the illness can be expected to progress.

The American Cancer Society provides an easy-to-understand description of the progressive phases of cancer using the TNM staging method.[13]

American Cancer Society Staging Criteria

Stage 0 Carcinoma in situ. Cancer is found only in the top lining of the bowel. This is the start-up phase of cancer.

Stage I Cancer has spread beyond the top lining of the bowel. It has entered and involves the inner layers of the bowel but is still confined to the bowel. Also called *Dukes' A colorectal cancer.*

Stage II Cancer has spread outside the bowel to nearby tissue, but not to the lymph nodes. Also called *Dukes' B colorectal cancer.*

Stage III Cancer has spread to nearby lymph nodes, but not to other parts of the body. Also called *Dukes' C colorectal cancer.*

Stage IV Cancer has spread to other parts of the body beyond the bowel. Also called *Dukes' D colorectal cancer.*

A cancer is called *carcinoma in situ* until it begins to invade the bowel wall. As the cancer expands beyond the surface tissue at the original site and reaches the inner layers of the bowel, it becomes an *invasive cancer*. The transformation from carcinoma in situ into invasive cancer is a slow process that can take several years.[14, 15]

Recurrent cancer refers to cancer that comes back after it has been treated, either to the original site or to another part of the body. There is a 20% to 40% probability for recurrence after colorectal-cancer treatment.[16]

Remission is the partial shrinkage or complete disappearance of cancer. It usually occurs as a result of treatment. Remission is a period when the disease seems to be under control. However, remission is not necessarily a cure. In general, five years without any trace of cancer is considered a cure.[17]

Pedunculated polyps are mushroom-shaped polyps with a stalk. They are considered less threatening than *sessile polyps*, flat polyps that develop directly from the bowel wall. Cancer spreading from the head of a pedunculated polyp must travel a greater distance before it reaches through the bowel wall and into the blood and lymph circulation systems.[18]

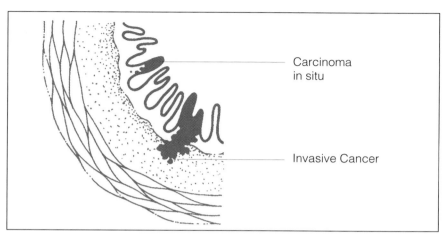

SESSILE POLYPS

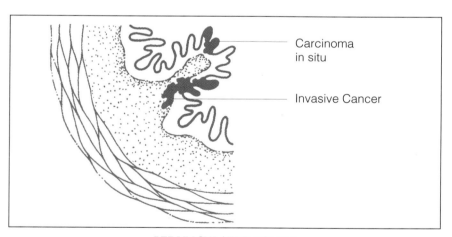

PEDUNCULATED POLYPS

Polyps Review: Common Terms and Definitions Used by Doctors and Medical Writers

The variety of terms used by doctors can be confusing. When my family doctor discovered rectal bleeding, he said that I probably had a "colonic polyp." The first specialist I saw used the word "adenoma." At Sloan-Kettering "neoplasm" seemed to be the most-popular description. It took some time before I realized that everybody was talking about the same thing. The following definitions will help you better understand what is going on and more easily communicate with your doctors. Also see Glossary, pages 231 to 243.

- A *polyp* is an abnormal growth that protrudes from the inner wall or lining of an organ such as the large bowel. The terms *polyp, tumor, neoplasm, neoplastic polyp, colonic polyp* and *lesion* are used interchangeably.

- Two types of polyps are generally found in the large bowel: *hyperplastic polyps* and *adenomatous polyps.*

- Small hyperplastic polyps are not considered to be dangerous.

- Adenomatous polyps, commonly referred to as *adenomas*, are larger and more dangerous. Upon discovery, they should be removed. Adenomas are believed to be the precursors (or predecessors) of colorectal cancer.

•Large-bowel tumors can be benign or malignant. Most newly discovered polyps are benign—5% to 10% will evolve into cancer. Current medical language tends to describe malignant growths with the terms *tumor* and *neoplasm.*

Polyp form, size, cell structure and stage of development are used to evaluate the cancerous potential of adenomas.

•*Pedunculated* and *sessile* describe the form of a polyp. Pedunculated polyps resemble a mushroom, complete with a stalk. The more-dangerous sessile polyps grow flat on the inner wall of the large bowel.

•The larger the polyp, the greater the risk of cancer. The danger zone for polyp size is considered to be 1 centimeter (1cm) in diameter. (1cm = .39 inch) Over 95% of malignancies develop in polyps larger than 1cm.

•*Villous, tubular* and *tubulovillous* are terms used to describe polyp-cell patterns as seen through a microscope. The cells of villous adenomas have a "shaggy" appearance. These are usually sessile polyps. About 20% of these adenomas contain cancer. The less-dangerous tubular adenomas have tube-like cells. Few of these contain cancer. Tubulovillous adenomas are comprised of elements of both cell-growth patterns.

•*Dysplasia* (pronounced dis-play-see-eh) is the abnormal development in size, shape and organization of cells which produce a growth. In essence, it is the 5- to 20-year transformation of benign polyps into malignancy. Dysplasia is usually described as being "mild" or "severe." It ends when the polyp is unquestionably malignant. The evolving of a benign polyp into cancer is sometimes called the *adenoma-carcinoma sequence*.

4

Screening Methods
EARLY DETECTION OF COLORECTAL CANCER

Screening is the search for a disease in an individual or a large group of people with no symptoms of that disease. The reason for screening is the same as that for having an annual physical examination: to detect medical problems at an early, controllable stage.

The goal of colorectal screening is the early discovery of adenomas or colorectal cancer and the timely removal of the suspicious growths. This greatly improves chances for patient survival. The three primary colorectal-screening procedures—digital rectal exam, stool-blood test and proctoscope examination—should be integral parts of the annual physical examination.

Digital rectal exam This is an examination of the anus and rectum by the physician's gloved and lubricated finger. The objective is to check the surface of the rectal wall for irregularly shaped or abnormally firm areas.[1] The physician also visually examines the fecal matter that comes out on the gloved finger to see if there is any blood.[2]

The digital rectal exam is also useful for detecting gynecological problems in women and prostate problems in men and should be an integral part of the annual physical examination for anyone over the age of 40.[3] The discovery of the adenoma in my colon was the direct result of finding traces of blood during this part of my annual physical.

Stool-blood test   It is usually recommended that the stool-blood test be performed annually after the age of 50.[4] The test requires thin smears from three consecutive bowel movements. These are collected by the patient at home and applied to chemically coated slides provided by the doctor. These slides are then sealed and returned to the doctor or a designated laboratory for analysis.[5] The stool-blood test is also called the *Fecal Occult Blood Test*, or *FOBT*. (The term *occult* means *hidden*.) The purpose of the test is to determine whether there is blood in the stool, which might occur for a variety of reasons. The test is *not* designed to detect cancer.[6]

Stool-blood tests are controversial because of scientific questions concerning accuracy, consistency and timeliness of laboratory processing.[7] The stool-blood test and the digital rectal exam are both less than ideal for the detection of blood in the digestive tract for several reasons:[8]

- Not all adenomas and cancers bleed.
- Not all adenomas and cancers bleed in sufficient quantity to show up on the tests.

•Bleeding can be intermittent and irregular. It can be missed during the time of the tests.

In other words: *patient, beware*. The person with a negative digital rectal exam or stool-blood test (no blood traces) must nevertheless remain on guard against developing a false sense of security.[9]

Sometimes the digital rectal exam or the stool-blood test will produce evidence of blood when there are no polyps or cancer. Bleeding may be caused by diet, such as rare meat in recent meals; by a reaction to various prescription and nonprescription drugs such as aspirin and vitamin-C pills; or by an unrelated medical problem such as hemorrhoids.[10] For these reasons patients are advised to refrain from eating red meat and taking pills for a couple of days before either test.

Almost 10% of "average-risk" people over the age of 50 will produce positive stool-blood tests.[11] Of this group, about 30% will actually have adenomas and 2% to 3% will have colorectal cancers.[12] The remainder and the great majority of the positive-test group will have no serious digestive-tract problems.[13]

Regardless of all the possible contradictions and accuracy difficulties, there can be no dispute that the digital rectal examination and stool-blood test are fast, easy, painless and inexpensive screening methods. They clearly increase the discovery rates of polyps and cancer. **Under all circumstances, tests showing the presence of blood must trigger immediate action to identify the reason.**

It is estimated that colorectal cancer cure rates of 85% or higher could be achieved if polyps were found and treated before they caused symptoms.[14] Although the stool-blood test and digital rectal exam are imperfect ways to detect colorectal cancer, no other cost-effective alternatives have been identified.[15]

Proctoscope (or "procto") examination   This procedure, more properly termed *proctosigmoidoscopy* (or *sigmoidoscopy*), involves the use of a fiberoptic, lighted-tube instrument called the *proctosigmoidoscope* (or *sigmoidoscope*). The sigmoidoscope is inserted through the anus into the rectum and into the lower parts of the colon, enabling the physician to perform a visual inspection of the lining of the lower bowel wall.[16] The purpose of the exam is to detect polyps in the anal canal, rectum and lower portions of the colon.

Two types of sigmoidoscopes are used for this exam: *rigid* and *flexible*. Most doctors now prefer the newer, flexible sigmoidoscope. Flexible sigmoidoscopes range from 35cm (about 12 inches) to 60cm (about 24 inches) in length. As patient and recipient of the sigmoidoscopy, do not be afraid to ask your doctor which type and size of scope is going to be used. I recommend you seek a doctor who utilizes the longer flexible instrument because it allows the inspection of a larger portion of the colon.[17] The out-dated rigid instrument is less accurate and causes considerably more discomfort to the patient.

It is generally recommended that a sigmoidoscopy be performed every 3 to 5 years after the age of 50.[18] The exam is relatively painless and does not require anesthesia. This allows the procedure to be performed in a doctor's office.[19]

The sigmoidoscope is commonly used to cut out a small sample of tissue from the inside of the large bowel so it can be examined by a laboratory. The procedure of removing tissue and its examination by a laboratory is called a *biopsy*. A biopsy can determine for certain whether the removed tissue is benign or malignant.

The flexible sigmoidoscope also has the capability of grasping and removing the entire polyp.[20] Whether a small piece of tissue or the entire polyp is removed, a biopsy will always be performed to see if cancer is present.

Some of the limitations of sigmoidoscopies plus alternative procedures are discussed in Chapter 7, Sigmoidoscopy versus Colonoscopy.

People at high risk for polyps or colorectal cancer (see page 13 for definition of *high risk*) should begin screening before age 40. They should also undergo more thorough screening than that provided by the three methods discussed above. In many cases, the diagnostic procedures discussed in Chapter 6, Diagnosis, should be considered routine screening methods for people classified as high risk.[21]

Colorectal-Cancer Screening
American Cancer Society Recommendations

Patient's Risk Category	Recommended Medical Procedure	Beginning Age	Frequency
Average risk	Digital rectal exam	40	Every year
	Fecal occult blood test	50	Every year
	Flexible sigmoidoscopy	50	Every 3-5 years
High Risk	Digital rectal exam	35-40	Every year
	Fecal occult blood test	35-40	Every year
	Colonscopy or Double-contrast barium enema	35-40	Every 3-5 years

5

Symptoms That Force Action
Your Body's Signals & What They Mean

Four of the most common digestive-system problems are *hemorrhoids, diverticulitis, polyps* and *colorectal cancer*. Hemorrhoids and diverticulitis, which are discussed in the Glossary, are usually not serious. The symptoms of the four disorders are similar, however, and may include:[1, 2, 3]

Bleeding Two warning signs that require an immediate visit to the doctor are the appearance of *any* amount of blood in the stool and a stool that is black in color.

Pain Some occasional abdominal discomfort is normal and is not necessarily indicative of cancer. Yet, if cramping or gnawing abdominal pain persists for over a week, particularly if it is associated with another symptom, there is good reason to seek medical advice.

Change in bowel habit   There is no standard for "normal bowel movement." Everyone is different. And day-to-day diet can affect anyone's bowel habits. However, when persistent diarrhea or constipation occurs, or when the two are alternating, these may be symptoms of a digestive-system problem, including polyps or cancer.

Tenesmus   This medical term describes an urgent and sometimes painful need to move one's bowels, coupled with a constant feeling of not being able to empty the rectum completely. It is an important symptom of rectal cancer.

Narrowing of stool   A thin, pencil-like stool is a signal of possible digestive-tract problems.

Unexplained weight loss, intermittent gas, lack of appetite, anemia, unusual paleness and fatigue   Any of these developments could be significant, especially when one or more of the other symptoms are also present.

In today's high-pressure world, symptoms of digestive-system disorders may seem inconsequential. We are often tempted to ignore the signals our bodies give us when something is wrong. In our culture, we also are often uncomfortable discussing matters dealing with excretion of body wastes. In addition, many polyps and early cancers fail to produce any symptoms whatsoever.

The advice is, *be aware!* Listen to your body. Follow your doctor's recommendations on screening tests appropriate for your age and risk level. Catching a disease in its early stages provides patients with a markedly better chance for a cure.

Never be concerned about overreacting or worry that you're wasting the doctor's time. I read many, many case histories while preparing this book and discovered an important theme. Repeatedly, patients described the agony of "looking back," of playing the "what-if" mind games that so often accompany serious illness. Ultimately, they held this common thought: "If only I'd had the good sense to get an early diagnosis, I would probably have avoided most of the despair, torment and heartbreak."

And, finally, do not accept the hyped-up claims of products advertising at-home treatment for stomach and digestion problems. When you consistently experience any of the symptoms described above, visit the doctor immediately for diagnosis. Any symptom that lasts more than two weeks should be considered a warning sign of a serious colorectal problem.

6

Diagnosis

COLONOSCOPY & BARIUM ENEMA AS DIAGNOSTIC TOOLS

When a sign or indication of an illness is identified, the medical effort shifts gears and becomes directed toward identifying (*diagnosing*) the problem. As previously detailed, the important signs may be discovered during a routine screening process (Chapter 4, Screening Methods) or by the patient's awareness of one or more of the common symptoms (Chapter 5, Symptoms That Force Action). When doctors suspect that colorectal cancer or polyps are present, the two procedures most commonly used for diagnostic purposes are the *colonoscopy* and the *double-contrast barium enema*.[1]

Colonoscopy The colonoscope is a fiberoptic, flexible, lighted, periscope-type instrument. It is 150cm (60 inches) long and no bigger in circumference than a finger. The colonoscope enables the physician to examine the entire length of the colon visually.

The procedure is very similar to a sigmoidoscopy, described in Chapter 4. Both are preceded by a thorough cleansing of the bowel as described later in this chapter. The major difference is that the colonoscope's greater length allows examining the entire length of the colon.[2]

Because anesthesia is required, the colonoscopy procedure usually takes place in a hospital on an out-patient basis. A typical stay in the hospital, from check-in to check-out, is several hours, although the colonoscopy itself takes about a half hour. Patients are exposed to a very slight risk of bowel perforation when undergoing a colonoscopy.[3, 4] Should this occur, the bowel is surgically repaired.

Polyps discovered during the course of a colonoscopy are removed through a procedure called a *polypectomy*. A wire loop is passed through the colonoscope and used to "lasso" the polyp.[5] An electrical charge is sent through the wire and the polyp is severed by cauterization. The process is practically painless and produces no after-effects.

If the shape, size or location of the growth makes it difficult to remove the entire polyp, the doctor will remove a piece of tissue from the growth to submit for biopsy.[6] A biopsy, which is also done when the whole growth is extracted, is the microscopic analysis of tissue to determine whether the tissue is benign or malignant.

Double-Contrast Barium Enema   Barium sulfate is a chalky substance that is given to the patient in enema form. It shows up clearly on X-rays, providing a silhouette of the large bowel and making possible the detection of growths in its surface.

Air is usually pumped into the bowel during the test to expand the bowel and make smaller tumors more visible. This technique is called an *air-contrast* or *double-contrast barium enema*.[7] In most colorectal diagnostic examinations, the double-contrast barium enema is utilized because it provides more dependable results than the traditional barium enema.[8]

To achieve maximum analytical results, both the colonoscopy and the double-contrast barium enema may be used. And, if for any reason it is impossible to perform a colonoscopy in searching for the source of potential colorectal problems, the *flexible sigmoidoscopy* can be used in conjunction with the double-contrast barium enema.[9]

Once the presence of malignant cells has been confirmed, the next diagnostic step is *staging* to determine to what extent the cancer has spread. For more information on staging, see Chapter 3, Polyp Form & the Spread of Cancer.

People of *average risk* (see page 14) should follow the routine screening regimens: digital rectal exam, stool-blood test and flexible sigmoidoscopy. However, there is no harm in the cautious person of average risk having a colonoscopy instead of a sigmoidoscopy sometime in the mid-50s, and every three to five years thereafter. A comparison of these two similar medical procedures is found in Chapter 7, Sigmoidoscopy versus Colonoscopy.

For anyone who has had colorectal cancer or polyps removed, it is recommended a follow-up colonoscopy be performed about one year later. This helps confirm that the first colonoscopy was entirely successful in removing all possible affected areas.[10] Thereafter, a colonoscopy at three- to five-year intervals is recommended. This is the amount of time it usually takes for growths to develop to the point where they can be detected.[11] Everyone should continue once-a-year surveillance with the digital rectal examination and stool-blood tests.

The National Cancer Institute's decade-long (1980 to 1990) National Polyp Study highlighted the life-saving value of colonoscopies. The 1,418 men who participated had previously had at least one precancerous adenoma removed. This made them more susceptible to developing new adenomas in the future. In fact, new polyps develop in nearly half of all people who have such growths removed.[12] Among the study's participants, the incidence of colorectal cancer was 76% to 90% less for those who received periodic colonoscopies than among those who did not.[13]

When a carcinoma (malignant growth) is found in the large bowel, there is a 30% risk of an adenomatous polyp and 2% risk of another carcinoma being present somewhere else in the large bowel.[14] The removal of adenomatous polyps has been projected to decrease the incidence of carcinomas by 85%.[15]

Some medical journals reluctantly list the *CEA assay* (*Carcinoembryonic Antigen Test*) as a diagnostic tool.[16] The CEA assay is a blood test that measures substances that may increase in the blood of a person with colorectal cancer. Because of different and fluctuating results, this is not a useful test as a screening or detection procedure. In fact, it may be of limited value in the diagnosis of colon cancer.[17] The CEA's main role is in monitoring a patient following treatment, when it may provide an early warning of cancer recurrence.[18]

Comparison of Colonoscopy & Double-Contrast Barium Enema

Diagnosis Colonoscopy is generally the preferred diagnostic method because polyps can be removed (or a biopsy performed) during the course of a colonoscopy. If abnormal growths are discovered with the double-contrast barium enema, the physician has to "go in" at a later time to remove them or to perform a biopsy (probably by employing a colonoscopy/polypectomy procedure).

Accuracy Both colonoscopy and the double-contrast barium enema are considered capable of producing, under optimum conditions, 90% to 95% accuracy for detecting abnormal growths (larger than 1cm) in the large bowel. Yet, uncertain procedural qualities, questionable standards and undependable evaluation methods have resulted in missing many more tumors when using the barium-enema procedure.

Smaller Growths Colonoscopy is generally recognized as being superior for detecting smaller growths (under 1cm). The smaller the growth, the less the risk of cancer.

Investigative Limits Both methods generally investigate the full length of the large bowel. In an estimated 1% to 15% of patients, the colonoscope has failed to reach the cecum, located at the beginning of the colon. (Refer to the illustration on page 41.)

Dangers Both procedures are universally considered to be safe. But, colonoscopy does carry a small risk of bowel perforation, which requires surgical repair. The danger of bowel perforation with the barium enema is somewhere in the 1 in 5000 range.

Personal Considerations Both procedures require the patient to clean out the bowel thoroughly the night before. Special diet, pills, liquids, enemas and/or suppositories are used to force bowel movements.

In a colonoscopy, the patient lies on his or her side (with knees bent up toward the chest) on an operating-room table. The physician, with one or more assistants, guides a small tube-like instrument into the anus and then up, through and around the colon. Sedation is required.

For a barium enema, the patient lies on a table under an X-ray machine. Sedation is not required. A tube is inserted into the bowel through the anus. Barium (a chalky liquid) and air are pumped into the large bowel and X-rays are taken from various positions. While a colonoscopy is rarely painful and carries a small danger of bleeding, the barium enema has no noticeable after-effects.

Representative Cost Ranges

	San Francisco, CA	Toledo, Ohio
Colonoscopy	$1700-$2000	$1600-$1900
Double-Contrast Barium Enema	$450-$600	$350-$500

7

Sigmoidoscopy versus Colonoscopy
UNDERSTANDING THE PROCEDURES

The flexible sigmoidoscope and colonoscope are similar in that they are both thin, flexible, fiberoptic instruments that allow the physician to see the internal "passageways" of the large bowel. The difference between them is their maximum extension limitations. The sigmoidoscope will go 30cm to 60cm (one to two feet) into a person (to the lower parts of the colon). The colonoscope is 150cm (five feet) long and allows the physician to investigate the entire large bowel, except in a few cases where the cecum is not reached.[1]

The use of the flexible sigmoidoscopy procedure illustrates the old adage, "Half a loaf of bread is better than no loaf." That is, the flexible sigmoidoscope will allow an examination of the lower end of the digestive tract but does not reach to the upper portions of the colon, where an estimated 30% to 50% of polyps and cancers are located.[2] Although there is dispute as to the actual number of polyps and cancers

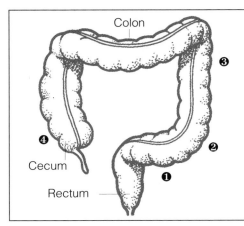

Colon	1 Extension limit of the rigid sigmoidoscope
	2 Extension limit of the flexible sigmoido-scope—35cm (14 in.)
	3 Extension limit of the flexible sigmoido-scope—60cm (24 in.)
Cecum	4 Extension limit of the flexible colonoscope
Rectum	

SIGMOIDOSCOPY VERSUS COLONOSCOPY

lodged in the upper colon, even the 30% estimate is large enough to cast doubts on the effectiveness of the sigmoi-doscopy procedure.[3]

In addition to its screening applications, the flexible sigmoidoscope is also widely employed in diagnosis. My personal experience was not uncommon. After blood was discovered during a routine digital rectal examination, my family physician sent me to a specialist, who performed a flexible sigmoidoscopy. I was then sent for a colonoscopy, to make sure all possible sources of blood had been identified. If I had been a more knowledgeable patient, I would not have undergone the limited sigmoidoscopy when there was going to be a thorough colonoscopy anyway. The sigmoidoscopy was an unpleasant, and essentially useless, procedure!

Another frightening possibility is that of a patient whose flexible sigmoidoscopy finds problems such as hemorrhoids in the anal canal or polyps in the lower colon. The patient believes his medical problems have been solved, only to discover later that there was also cancer in the upper colon, the area not investigated by the flexible sigmoidoscopy.

An Indiana University School of Medicine study included 210 average-risk physicians, dentists and their spouses.[4] The participants, all between 60 and 75 years of age, had experienced no symptoms of colorectal problems and had no close family histories of colorectal disorders. In addition, to qualify for the test group all participants had to have negative stool-blood tests for three successive days during the week before the study commenced.

Each participant was given a colonoscopy. Results showed 53 subjects (25%) had adenomatous polyps, 18 had harmless hyperplastic polyps, and 2 had cancer. One of the cancers and approximately 50% of the adenomas were located in the upper colon areas. If the flexible sigmoidoscopy had been used instead of the colonoscopy, 50% of the adenomas and cancers would have gone undetected.[5]

Knowing half the story via sigmoidoscopy is certainly better than knowing nothing. But the person interested in learning whether colorectal problems are developing inside his or her body would logically choose the more thorough colonoscopy. Using a flexible sigmoidoscope to examine a relatively small part of the potential problem area is like undergoing screening for lung cancer by taking an X-ray of one lung.

The argument supporting sigmoidoscopies is that they are relatively easy, fast procedures that can be accomplished in a doctor's office, at a lower price. The procedure is not inexpensive, however. Average costs usually range from $500 to $900. The cost for a colonoscopy, usually performed in a hospital on an outpatient basis, is even higher, ranging from $1,200 to $2,000.

Medical insurance does not cover the colonoscopy as a screening procedure when there are no signs of a colorectal problem. Medical-insurance companies differ in their approach to paying for a sigmoidoscopy as a screening process. Of course, once there is an indication of colorectal problems, almost all insurance companies will pay for both procedures. In fact, my insurance company paid for a flexible sigmoidoscopy and then *two* colonoscopies—the first to remove the head of the adenomatous polyp and the second a month later to remove the polyp's stalk, accidentally missed on the first try.

8

Treatment
AFTER CANCER HAS BEEN IDENTIFIED

The optimum objective for treatment is the fast and complete removal of the tumor. If it is an adenoma or early (Stage 0) carcinoma in situ (see Glossary for definitions), the growth will often be removed without cutting the skin. The doctor enters the large bowel through the anus and performs either a *polypectomy*, for mushroom-like pedunculated growths, or a *local excision*, surgical removal of a flat, sessile-type polyp and surrounding tissue.[1] (See Chapter 3, Polyp Form & the Spread of Cancer, for illustrations and a discussion of polyps. See Chapter 6, Diagnosis, for a description of a polypectomy.) The patient should not experience any side effects from these minor surgical procedures. If the cancer has not spread, the polypectomy or local excision will most likely be the cure.

For more advanced colorectal disorders, there are four primary treatments:[2]

- Surgery
- Radiation
- Chemotherapy
- Biological Therapy (Immunotherapy)

Once the location and stage of the cancer have been determined, an individual treatment strategy will be devised, taking into account the patient's age and general health as well as his or her probable reactions to the available treatment methods. (See Chapter 3, Polyp Form & the Spread of Cancer, for an explanation of staging.)

Surgery   Surgery is the most-often-used treatment and will cure approximately 50% of colorectal-cancer patients.[3] Of course, the potential for success greatly depends on how much the disease has spread at the time of the initial diagnosis.

Although radical, emergency and innovative surgical strategies exist, the most common surgery involves cutting out the section of the bowel containing the cancer, usually removing some of the surrounding tissue and the nearby lymph nodes as well. A pathologist's examination of the additional tissue and lymph nodes will provide an indication as to whether the cancer has spread.

If possible, the surgeon will reattach the two unconnected ends of the bowel. This achieves the same result as splicing two electrical wires together—just as electrical current can flow through a spliced wire, a person can resume

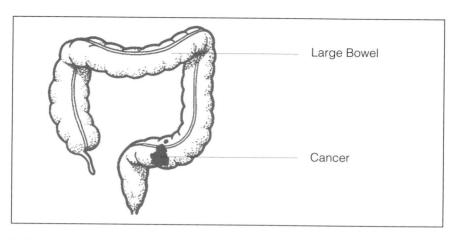

Large Bowel

Cancer

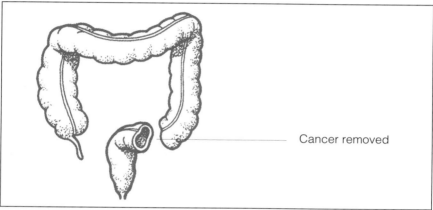

Cancer removed

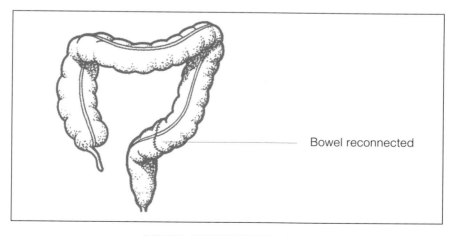

Bowel reconnected

BOWEL-RESECTION SURGERY

normal bowel movement through a bowel that has been rejoined after removal of a cancerous section.[4] The term used for the surgical removal of cancer and the rejoining of the bowel is *bowel resection*. The step of reconnecting the two ends of the bowel is *anastomosis*.[5]

In those rare situations where the ends of the bowel cannot immediately be rejoined, a *colostomy* is performed. The surgeon creates an opening called a *stoma* in the abdomen wall.[6] The normal excretion functions of the large bowel are bypassed and body waste is automatically eliminated via the stoma into a special bag called an *appliance*.[7] The appliance, which sticks to the skin with a special glue, is thrown away after it is used. It does not show under clothing and most people are able to take care of the appliances by themselves. There are no nerve endings in the stoma and therefore the colostomy is not a source of pain.[8]

A colostomy is usually a temporary condition. After some bowel healing has occurred, the procedure can be reversed. The two sections of the bowel are rejoined and normal bowel functions are regained.[9]

In some advanced-stage cancers and for cancers located very close to the anus, the colostomy will be permanent. The number of permanent colostomies is steadily decreasing, thanks to earlier detection and improved treatment methods. After overcoming initial emotional and physical problems, patients who undergo a permanent colostomy should be able to lead normal and active lives.[10]

A colostomy is one type of *ostomy*,[11] the medical term used to describe any surgically created opening in the body. For the patient confronting a colostomy, the American Cancer Society distributes an insightful, comprehensive and easy-to-understand report entitled *Colostomy—A Guide* (publication #4703). See Chapter 10, Information Resources for the Colorectal-Cancer Patient, for American Cancer Society contact information.

Radiation   *Radiation* therapy, also called *X-ray therapy, radiotherapy, cobalt treatment* or *irradiation*, employs penetrating, high-energy rays to kill and eliminate cancer cells and to prevent cancer cells from growing and dividing.[12] Radiation may be used before an operation to reduce the cancer cells, and during or after an operation to destroy malignant cells not removed by the surgery. Patients usually obtain radiation therapy as outpatients in hospitals, clinics or private medical offices.[13]

Endocavitary irradiation uses an X-ray tube fitted onto a scope. This is inserted through the anus. By looking through the scope, the doctor can see the inside of the rectum and aim radiation directly at the tumor.[14]

Radiation usually refers to *external radiation,* meaning a machine outside the body aims rays at the affected area.

Internal radiation is a general term referring to the surgical implanting of radiation via tubes, wires or seeds on or next to the tumor.[15]

Chemotherapy   *Chemotherapy* uses drugs that destroy cancer cells by interfering with their growth or by preventing their reproduction.[16] It may be given to patients in pill form or by injection into a muscle, an artery or a vein. The drugs travel through the bloodstream to almost every area of the body. Depending on which drugs are used, the patient may have to stay in the hospital for a few days so the effects of the drugs can be evaluated and doses regulated. From then on, the patient may be given chemotherapy as an outpatient, in a medical office or at home. Chemotherapy is most often given in a cycle: a treatment period followed by a rest period, then another treatment and so on.[17]

One of the most common drugs used for fighting colorectal cancer is *5-fluorouracil* (or *5-FU*).[18] Although there is no proof that chemotherapy improves survival, 5-FU provides short-term relief for 20% to 25% of patients with advanced disease.[19] An experimental chemotherapy uses a small pump to deliver drugs directly to the liver, the most common site of colorectal-cancer spread.[20]

Radiation and Chemotherapy Side Effects Both radiation and chemotherapy treatments can produce side effects. Because cancer can spread and destroy, the treatments used to combat this potentially lethal disease must be powerful. It is rarely possible to limit the effects so that only cancer cells are destroyed. Some healthy cells are damaged at the same time, causing unpleasant side effects.

Radiation therapy commonly causes skin reactions such as redness or dryness in the area being treated. Other side effects include fatigue, diarrhea, nausea and vomiting.[21]

The side effects of chemotherapy depend on the drugs that are given and the individual response of the patient. Chemotherapy commonly affects hair cells, blood-forming cells and cells lining the digestive tract. As a result, patients may have side effects such as hair loss, lowered blood counts, nausea or vomiting. Most side effects end after the treatment is over.[22]

Loss of appetite is a serious problem for some cancer patients. Researchers are learning that patients who eat well are better able to withstand the side effects of treatment. Therefore, nutrition is an important part of any treatment plan. Eating well primarily means getting enough calories to prevent weight loss and having enough protein in the diet to build and repair skin, hair, muscles and organs. Many patients find that eating small meals throughout the day is easier than eating three large meals.[23]

The roles of radiation and chemotherapy in colorectal-cancer treatment have not yet been conclusively determined. Extensive research continues to try to define the best methods to maximize benefits while minimizing side effects.

Dealing with cancer treatments is further discussed in Appendix B, Using Good Nutrition to Combat Cancer Treatment Side Effects. The National Cancer Institute (NCI) distributes two excellent publications entitled *Radiation Therapy and You: A Guide to Self-Help During Treatment* and *Chemotherapy and You: A Guide to Self-Help During Treatment*. NCI contact information may be found in Chapter 10, Information Resources for the Colorectal-Cancer Patient.

Biological Therapy   *Biological therapy*, also called *immunotherapy*, encourages a person's own body to fight the cancer. This newest type of cancer treatment uses materials made by the body or fabricated in a laboratory to boost, direct and restore the natural defenses against disease. Scientists have identified a number of substances called *biological-response modifiers (BRMs)* that may trigger or stimulate the body's immune system to fight cancer.[24]

Although scientists have known about biological-response modifiers for years, it is extremely difficult to isolate and purify them. In addition to inhibiting cancer-cell growth directly, BRMs may also:[25]

- enhance the immune system's ability to fight cancer-cell growth.
- eliminate, regulate or suppress body responses that permit cancer growth.
- stimulate a cancer cell to transform into a less harmful cell or into a normal cell.
- block the process that changes a normal or pre-cancerous cell into a cancerous cell.
- enhance the body's ability to repair normal cells damaged by chemotherapy or radiation.

Many substances are currently under evaluation. For colorectal cancer, the most-often used biological-response modifiers are *levamisole* and *interleukin-2 (IL-2)*.[26]

Adjuvant therapy Adjuvant therapy is the use of secondary treatments to enhance the effectiveness of the primary treatments.[27] In March 1994 Sloan-Kettering Cancer Center reported: "With a combination of high dose radiation and chemotherapy administered before surgery, Sloan-Kettering physicians have been able to avoid permanent colostomies in many patients who previously would have required this radical procedure." In this case, surgery was the *primary* treatment while radiation and chemotherapy were *adjuvant* therapies.

From a historical standpoint, adjuvant therapy is usually given after the primary treatment, when all known cancer has been removed but when there is still a risk of hidden cancer cells remaining. It is given with the expectation of decreasing the chance of cancer recurrence.[28]

There is a 20% to 40% risk of recurrence after successful colorectal cancer surgery. And, there is a 2% to 10% risk that a totally new cancer will appear after such surgery.[29] Adjuvant therapy may be referred to as *adjuvant chemotherapy, adjuvant radiation* or *adjuvant biological therapy* to indicate which form of secondary treatment is being utilized.

Palliative treatment   *Palliative treatment* is the use of medical remedies to relieve pain, control symptoms or prevent complications, as opposed to instituting a cure. It may include any of the cancer treatments described in this chapter. The underlying objective is to improve the patient's quality of life. In advanced cancer situations, palliative treatment is primarily aimed at comforting the patient.[30]

Treatment Follow-up   Surgery is applicable in about 85% of colorectal-cancer cases and cures about 50% of such cases.[31] The main goal of follow-up procedures is early detection of recurrent tumors, which appear after surgery in 20% to 40% of patients.[32, 33]

No set rules or guidelines govern a doctor's follow-up procedures. However, results of recent surveys indicate that most surgeons take over surveillance rather than sending patients back to their primary doctors.[34]

This surveillance usually consists of office visits for examinations every 3 to 6 months for about three years after the operation. For the next few years, visits are required every 6 to 12 months. Follow-up procedures generally cover only a five-year period because five years without a recurrence of cancer is usually considered a cure.[35]

One test utilized in the follow-up examinations is the *CEA assay (Carcinoembryonic Antigen Test)*. This is a blood test that measures a substance in the blood that could rise as a result of cancer. Although questions exist as to its reliability, it is often used after cancer treatment because a rise in a patient's CEA level could be the first sign of cancer recurrence.[36, 37]

Rectal-surgery patients should expect to have a sigmoidoscopy as part of almost every doctor's appointment and a colonoscopy about a year after surgery. Additional colonoscopies should occur at 2- to 3-year intervals.[38]

Colon-cancer patients will often have a colonoscopy a year after surgery. If it is negative, colonoscopies will normally be required at 2- to 3-year intervals for the next four years. Depending on the individual patient's history and the doctor's personal opinion, additional follow-up strategies may include chest X-rays, CT scans, liver-function tests, barium enemas and various blood tests.[39]

Clinical Trials:
A Different and Added Perspective To Treatment

Treating colorectal cancer is not an exact science and no clear-cut solutions exist. Yet, because of colorectal cancer's widespread attack on so many unsuspecting people, well-organized, never-ending *clinical trials* continue to make advances on fighting this disease. They deal with all aspects of prevention, detection and treatment. Broadly speaking, clinical trials can be defined as closely monitored research studies using patients.[40]

Patients usually take part in clinical trials with the hope of benefiting from the newest medical advances. Doctors conduct clinical trials to find out whether new treatments are safe and more effective than current methods. The risks of being part of a clinical trial are limited because the testing of cancer treatments on humans begins only after long, intensive laboratory and animal studies. Unfortunately, new cancer treatments are rare. Most clinical trials involve testing refinements to standard treatments.

One positive by-product of participating in a clinical trial is that the patient receives an added degree of expert monitoring and supervision.[41] It is a form of "add-on" alternative treatment that warrants careful consideration and review with doctors.[42] All doctors treating cancer should be knowledgeable about theories and specifics of clinical trials. Further information on clinical trials is in Appendix G. The National Cancer Institute (1-800-4-CANCER) also maintains relevant information about many current clinical trials.

If you are considering taking part in a clinical trial, the following questions may supply some important answers.

- What is the purpose of this study?
- Who is sponsoring it?
- What does the study involve? What kinds of tests and treatments are included?
- What is the standard treatment I will receive if I do not participate in the trial?
- What is likely to happen to me without any treatment?
- What are the advantages and disadvantages of the standard treatment?
- What are the advantages and disadvantages of the clinical-trial treatment?
- What is the theory that the trial is expected to prove? What is the hoped-for result?
- How could the trial treatment affect my daily life?
- What side effects could I expect from all treatments?
- How long will the study last?
- Is hospitalization required? If so, for how long and how often?
- What are the costs? Will treatments be free?
- If the treatment proves harmful, what treatment will the study make available to me?
- What type of follow-up care is part of the study?
- In addition to trial treatments, are any other responsibilities required, such as doctor visits, completing paperwork, interviews, etc.?

9

Prognosis
LOOKING TO THE FUTURE

The terms in *italics* have been previously explained in the text and are also defined in the Glossary.

Prognosis is the medical prediction as to what course an illness will follow in the future. When the patient is told that he or she has *colorectal cancer*—this is a *diagnosis*. When the patient is told his or her chances for a complete cure—that is the prognosis.

For people diagnosed with *benign adenometous polyps* (*adenomas*), the prognosis is complete cure when the adenomas are detected and removed early. If they are not removed, there is a risk that benign polyps will slowly evolve into *cancer* during the next 5 to 20 years.[1] In fact, about 1 in 10 adenomas will become *malignant*.[2] Thus, the early removal of the adenomas can be expected to lower the danger of colorectal cancer.

However, once *polyps* are discovered, the "die has been cast." The patient must realize that he or she is in a *high-risk* category, and surveillance will be required for the rest of his or her life. After polyps are removed, there is a 50% chance that new polyps will appear sometime in the future.[3]

The prognosis and *treatment* for colorectal cancer depend on how far the disease has spread before being detected, the depth of penetration and the extent of *lymph-node* involvement.[4] Secondary factors include location, size, form of tumor (*pedunculated* or *sessile*), *cell* type (*tubular* or *villous*) and the patient's age, general health and reactions to treatments.[5, 6]

Differences exist when comparing cancer in the *colon* and cancer in the *rectum*. But it is possible to provide general guidelines for treatment and accompanying prognosis for colorectal cancer by following *staging* criteria.[7, 8, 9]

Colorectal Cancer Treatment and Prognosis

The significance of the term "5-year survival rate" is that a patient is usually considered cured if no further symptoms have appeared five years after treatment.[10]

Stage 0 5-year survival rate: 95% to 100% [11, 12]

Definition: Start up, non-invasive *carcinoma in situ* has not spread beyond the lining of the *large bowel*.
Treatment:[13, 14, 15, 16]
- *Polypectomy*
- *Local excision*
- *Wedge resection*
- *Bowel resection* and *anastomosis* (for large tumors)
- Electrocoagulation, electrofulguration (for rectal cancer)
- *Radiation, endocavitary irradiation* (for rectal cancer)

Stage I (or Dukes' A)—5-year survival rate: 75% to 100% [17, 18]

Definition: Cancer is still confined to the large bowel, but has spread deeper into the large bowel.

Treatment: At any stage, *bowel resection* and *anastomosis* are the preferred and primary treatments. Whenever cancer is situated in the rectum, too close to the anus, it might be impossible to perform resection. Regardless of the stage, this condition can force either a temporary or permanent *colostomy*. Electrofulguration, electrocoagulation or *endocavitary irradiation* could be utilized in selected cases. [19, 20, 21] *Radiation* could be a either a primary or an adjuvant treatment for Stage I rectal cancer. *Chemotherapy* is sometimes used as an adjuvant rectal-cancer treatment. [22, 23]

Stage II (or Dukes' B)—5-year survival rate: 50% to 75% [24, 25]

Definition: Cancer has spread outside the large bowel to nearby *tissue*, but has not yet reached the lymph nodes.

Treatment: *Surgical resection* and *anastomosis* are the preferred primary treatments. When the tumor is in the rectum, near the anus, there is a chance that a temporary or permanent colostomy could be required. The Stage II patient is a candidate for *radiation* or *chemotherapy adjuvant treatments* used separately or in combination before and after surgery. [26, 27] Radiation is sometimes used during surgery. [28] *Biological therapy* combined with *chemotherapy* is now being evaluated as a Stage II treatment. [29]

Stage III (Dukes' C)—5-year survival rate: 30% to 50% [30, 31]

Definition: Cancer has spread beyond the large bowel and has reached the lymph nodes, but has not yet spread to other parts of the body.

Treatment: *Bowel resection* and *anastomosis* are the preferred and primary treatments. Recent studies have supported the theory that the number of lymph nodes involved impacts on prognosis and treatment. Patients with fewer than four affected lymph nodes have the best chance for a cure.[32] It is understandable that much research focuses on Stage III in an attempt to devise treatments to stop the spread of cancer before it reaches the serious, less-treatable Stage IV.

5-Fluorouracil, commonly called *5-FU*, is the standard *chemotherapy* drug. It may be used by itself or in combination with other therapies.[33] Studies have shown that a combination of *adjuvant* chemotherapy and *biological therapy* (*levamisole*) can reduce the risk of dying from Stage III disease by about 33%. It may also reduce the risk of cancer *recurrence*.[34]

When the tumor is in the rectum or near the anus, or when there is extensive cancer spreading throughout the large bowel, there is a greater chance that a temporary or permanent colostomy will be required. *Radiation* before, during and after operations (by itself or in combination with chemotherapy) has been used as adjuvant treatment.[35] Also, biological therapy by itself (or in combination with other therapies) has shown limited success in Stage III colorectal-cancer treatments.[36, 37]

Stage IV (Dukes' D)—5-year survival rate: 0% to 30% [38, 39]

Definition: Cancer has spread beyond the large bowel to
other parts of the body. About 50% of patients diagnosed with *colorectal cancer* will eventually die of
metastatic disease that appears somewhere else in the
body.[40] In about 25% of newly diagnosed colorectal-
cancer patients the cancer has already spread to other
parts of the body.[41] In colorectal-cancer patients, metastasis occurs most often in the liver, appearing there in
about 35% of these patients. The lungs are the second
most common site of colorectal-cancer metastasis.[42]

Treatment: Unlike treatments for the other stages of colorectal cancer where the key objective is curing the
disease, Stage IV goals often deal with *palliative treatment* to relieve pain and generally provide for a better
quality of life. Even if the cancer cannot be cured,
bowel resection and *anastomosis* are the preferred and
primary treatments to guard against suffering caused
by such major problems as obstruction, bleeding and
bowel perforation.[43] Sometimes *resection* and *anastomosis* are performed to make the colon go around the cancer so the colon can still function.[44]

A majority of colorectal-cancer deaths can be attributed to liver complications. If there is isolated, definitive liver metastasis, the same surgery can possibly
remove the colon and liver diseases.[45] Survival chances
can be increased 18% to 40% if the infected parts of the
liver can be surgically removed.[46] Surgery can also be

undertaken to remove the infected parts of the other organs such as the lungs or ovaries.[47] *Chemotherapy* (5-FU) is often considered standard treatment that can provide relief for about 20% to 25% of the patients.[48] All forms of therapies—by themselves or in combinations—are used for treatment purposes. Laser therapy has been used in attempts to reduce the bulk of a tumor causing an obstruction and/or to stop bleeding.[49]

Recurrent Colorectal Cancer

Definition: *Recurrent cancer* is cancer that reappears after successful treatment and a period when there is no evidence of cancer. There is 20% to 40% chance that surgically removed colorectal cancer will reappear either in the large bowel or somewhere else in the body.[50] There is a higher risk for recurrence of rectal cancer than of colon cancer. There is a 2% to 10% chance for developing a new cancer in the colon or rectum. In about 80% of the cases, recurrent colorectal cancer is detected within two years after surgery.[51]

Treatment: Although recurrent colorectal cancer carries a poor prognosis, surgery provides the best chance for long-term survival.[52] The first question to ask when confronted with recurrent colorectal cancer is, "Can surgery be performed?" Treatment ultimately depends on the location and penetration of the disease and the age and health of the patient.[53] There are no standard treatments for recurrent colorectal cancer.[54] In situations where there is only one well-defined recurrence such as in the large bowel or liver and surgery is possible, the tumor is removed and there is a good chance for survival.[55] Sometimes, the cancer will return only where sections of the bowel have been sewn together. Such suture-line recurrences can be surgically removed with improved chances for cure.[56] Recurrent cancer is often analyzed in the same context as Stage IV cancer and the same treatments are applicable.[57]

Prognosis Conclusions: Early Detection

This chapter began by identifying survival rates of near 100% for start-up colorectal cancer and survival rates of 0% to 30% for the advanced disease. If nothing else, the startling disparity in these survival percentages should drive home the importance of early detection.

More than 46,000 Minnesota residents participated in a 13-year program aimed at measuring the effectiveness of early detection of bowel disorders.[58] Utilizing the *fecal occult test (FOBT)* as the initial *screening* procedure, researchers found 33% fewer deaths in the group using the fecal occult tests. The lower death rate was directly attributed to the effective treatments of colorectal cancer and polyps detected in an early stage.

Some people avoid the routine screening procedure and/or delay following up on *symptoms* of colorectal cancer. They may be worried about the discomfort and embarrassment that accompanies rectal exams or they may fear that the detection of cancer will lead to ugly, extensive surgery.

The fact is: **Early detection reduces the likelihood for major surgery and greatly reduces the life-threatening danger of colorectal cancer.**

Early detection is the cornerstone of colorectal-cancer prognosis. When dealing with colorectal cancer, a person's survival very often depends on his or her actions in responding to symptoms and in following through with annual physical examinations. When detected early and treated promptly, colorectal cancer is one of the most curable of all diseases.

10

Information Resources for the Colorectal-Cancer Patient
WHERE TO LOOK FOR HELP

The National Cancer Institute (NCI)—1-800-4-CANCER

The National Cancer Institute is a division of the National Institutes of Health (NIH). An agency of the federal government, NCI performs two main functions. First is research into cancer prevention, diagnosis and treatment. Second is the supplying of cancer-related information to the public. All NCI services are free.

The NCI's **Cancer Information Service (CIS)** is a nationwide telephone network for patients, their family and friends, and health-care professionals. CIS specialists have extensive training in providing up-to-date and understandable information about cancer. They can answer questions in English and Spanish, and can send free printed material on request. In addition, CIS offices serve specific geographic areas and have information about cancer-related services and resources in each region. Their toll-free number is 1-800-4-CANCER (1-800-422-6237).

NCI publishes an immense amount of cancer-related literature that anybody can get by calling the Cancer Information Service. Many pamplets relating to colorectal cancer are listed in the Bibliography, pages 244 to 251. Booklets of a more general nature include the following:

What You Need To Know About . . . This is a series of booklets about different types of cancer. Specify a primary cancer site (such as colon or rectum) in your request.

Radiation Therapy and You: A Guide To Self-Help During Treatment. Radiation therapy, its goals and side effects, and helpful suggestions to patients are discussed.

Chemotherapy and You: A Guide To Self-Help During Treatment. Provides detailed information about how chemotherapy is used in cancer treatment and how to manage the side effects of drug treatment.

Questions and Answers About Pain Control. Discusses various medical and nonmedical methods of pain control.

Answers to Your Questions About Metastatic Cancer. Presents information about what happens when cancer spreads.

Taking Time. Support for People With Cancer and the People Who Care About Them. Discusses the special emotional and personal problems faced by people with cancer.

The Cancer Information Service can also access the **Physicians Data Query (PDQ)** computer system, which provides up-to-date information on cancer. The PDQ data base is updated with the assistance of more than 400 cancer health professionals in the United States.

CancerNet is a way to obtain PDQ information using Internet electronic mail.

CancerFax (fax number: 1-301-402-5874) can be accessed 24 hours a day, 7 days a week. It provides information from the PDQ.

Appendix E, beginning on page 211, is an explanation of NCI's Community Clinical Oncology Program. Appendix F, beginning on page 213, is an explanation of NCI's Cancer Centers Program. Appendix G, beginning on page 220, explains NCI's Clinical Trials Cooperative Group program, with a corresponding list of associated medical facilities. NCI's address is:

> National Cancer Institute
> Building 31, Room 10A24
> 9000 Rockville Pike
> Bethesda, MD 20892

American Cancer Society (ACS)—1-800-ACS-2345

The American Cancer Society is a national organization comprised of over two million volunteers. The ACS is dedicated to fighting cancer through research, education, service and rehabilitation programs. Telephones are answered by trained volunteers, many of whom have had cancer themselves. Both local and headquarters offices are prepared to supply a wealth of information on every aspect of cancer. Additionally, the ACS carries on a wide ranging effort of patient/family services. The list of ACS chartered divisions is in Appendix D, beginning on page 206. The address of the national headquarters is:

American Cancer Society, Inc.
1599 Clifton Road N.E.
Atlanta, GA 30329

United Ostomy Association—1-800-826-0826

The United Ostomy Association is organized and administered by people with ostomies. An *ostomy* is a surgically created opening in the body. A *colostomy* is one of several different kinds of ostomies. This organization is dedicated to helping ostomy patients return to normal life through mutual aid and emotional support. The address is:

United Ostomy Association
36 Executive Park, Suite 120
Irvine, CA 92714

11

Patient Questions
"KNOWLEDGE IS SALVATION" (SOCRATES)

Several years ago, posters with the following message were sent by the National Cancer Institute to cancer centers throughout the United States to be placed in patient waiting areas.

Notice to Patients

To obtain maximum benefit from your treatment, become a partner with your physician. You should understand everything being done for you and how and why it works. To do this you must ask questions! Your doctor wants you to understand, but will not know your concerns unless you express them. A physician or nurse will take as much time as necessary to explain anything about your condition that you do not understand. A partnership like this will ensure that the care you receive is optimal.

Previous chapters have provided general information to help you understand the disease known as *colorectal cancer*. Questions in this chapter are designed to help shed light on your own individual situation. Patient education is a key component in the battle against colorectal cancer.

Coping with illness and dealing with doctors is not easy for any of us. Normally self-confident people become tongue-tied and submissive. But this is a time to overcome fears and become assertive. Do not allow unanswered questions to further distress a mind that is already overwhelmed with worry and fear. Do not be intimidated by doctors who give the impression that conversations and explanations impose on their busy schedules.

At some point you will find yourself in the uneasy situation when the doctor must explain the seriousness of the illness. You will struggle to keep your composure while putting up a brave front. The doctor will explain that it is important that you fully understand the medical dilemma. Yet, in the back of everyone's mind is the knowledge that time is limited. Other patients are waiting and the doctor must move on despite your feelings and need for reassurance and comfort.

Think through your questions before entering the doctor's office. Write your questions down. Otherwise you may well forget half of them. Take a notebook to the appointment to write down the answers. Some patients bring cassette recorders with them. Fear and anxiety can naturally lead to "selective hearing," making it difficult for the patient to remember all that was said. With a tape of the meeting, the conversation can be played back as many times as necessary to catch all the details.

Whenever the doctor supplies an answer that you don't completely understand, stop the conversation and ask for a better explanation. You might say to the doctor, "Let me repeat what you've just said to make sure I understood correctly."

It is also a good idea to ask a family member or good friend to go with you to the doctor. He or she can provide another viewpoint, ask additional questions and listen to and explain the doctor's answers. This also serves as a means of sharing information about your illness with family and friends. They can better understand your situation and help with decisions.

I have found that many doctors are good about returning telephone calls, usually at the end of the day. An organized patient working from a prepared list of questions can usually obtain good, to-the-point answers during such calls. The smart patient must be sensitive to overkill and keep such calls to a minimum.

It is likely that one of two unexpected—and frightening—developments will have started you asking questions. Either your doctor told you that the routine screening tests indicated there might be a digestive-system problem. (See Chapter 4, Screening Methods.) Or, you recognized one of the danger signals, such as blood in the stool. (See Chapter 5, Symptoms That Force Action.)

With either of these sudden occurrences, you are thrust into a strange reality of new priorities. You are about to embark on the diagnosis experience, where the all-too-real possibility exists that a potentially life-threatening condition will be discovered.

The launching of the diagnostic effort is often the patient's first exposure to medical testing. The first objective of the tests is to identify the source of the problem. In the case of suspected colorectal cancer this will be done with either a colonoscopy or a double-contrast barium enema. (See Chapter 6, Diagnosis)

Patient questions concerning these or any other medical tests could include:

- What is the full name of the test?
- What is the purpose of the test?
- Why do you recommend the test?
- What will happen to me during the test?
- What type of results can be expected?
- What happens if the test is negative and shows no trace of illness?
- What are the next steps if the test is positive?
- How long will it take to get the results?
- How long does it take to perform this test?
- Do I need to take the test in the hospital?
- If "yes," how long will I be in the hospital?
- Are preparations required before I take the test?
- Will I have any after-effects?
- If "yes," what are they? How long will they last?
- Is the test painful?
- What will it cost?

The next step in the diagnosis process is determined by the test results. The best-case scenario is the discovery of a non-serious ailment, such as hemorrhoids or diverticulitis.

These can be easily treated and quickly cured.

Second best is the detection of benign polyps or beginning cancer, called *carcinoma in situ*. These can usually be removed and cured with minor surgery procedures, such as a polypectomy or local excision. (See Chapter 8, Treatment.)

A third possibility is that the diagnostic tests will show no abnormal growths or are inconclusive. This *could* mean that the original symptoms or screening procedures were incorrect. However, if symptoms persist or screening continues to produce positive results, you must resume testing. The underlying problem must be identified before stopping the testing.

The worst-case scenario is the discovery of cancer. Whatever your state of mind prior to this point, the word "cancer" automatically evokes a sullen and serious despair. The reality of having cancer produces an ever-expanding flow of questions. Ask them all. There is no such thing as a "dumb" question!

The first question that usually creeps into the mind is, "Am I going to die?" The answer is, "Yes, eventually. But probably not from cancer." It's much too early in the diagnosis process to provide any predictions and, in any case, the chances of dying from cancer today are dramatically less than ever before.

To confirm the diagnosis of cancer, a *biopsy* is performed. Tissue is extracted from a suspicious area and sent to a pathologist who conducts a microscopic examination. The examination determines whether the tissue is *benign* or *malignant*. When advising a patient of the presence of cancer, the doctor's key source for information is the pathology report. It will also provide the basis for cancer-related decisions in the future. At this point, a patient's questions might include:

- Have you (the doctor) personally talked to the pathologist?
- Has the report been reviewed by another pathologist?
- Is it possible to get a copy of the pathologist's report?
- Should we send the tissue slides to another pathologist for an independent opinion?
- If the answer is "no," why not?
- If the answer is "yes," the patient should then ask the doctor to make the arrangements.

With the diagnosis of cancer, the doctor usually begins a staging process to determine how far the cancer has spread. (See Chapter 3, Polyp Form & the Spread of Cancer.) When diagnosis and staging are complete, the doctor is normally ready to recommend treatment. Questions to ask at this time might include:

- Where is the cancer located?
- How big is the cancer?
- What stage is the cancer?
- Has the cancer spread?
- If "yes," to what other parts of the body?
- If "I don't know," how will you go about finding out if it has spread? And, how long will it take for you to find out if it has spread?

- Will the treatment cure my cancer?
- If "yes," how long should it take before I am cured?
- If "I don't know," on a scale of 1 to 10, with 10 being a complete cure, what is your educated guess as to my chances of getting completely cured?
- If "no," why am I taking this treatment?

In the case of colorectal cancer, the patient will, in all likelihood, be presented with one, or a combination, of four different treatments: surgery, radiation therapy, chemotherapy or biological therapy (immunotherapy). (See Chapter 8, Treatment.)

Surgery is the preferred and most-used treatment—about 50% of colorectal-cancer cases are cured with an operation, usually a bowel resection. The patient's questions regarding surgery should include:

- Why should I have surgery instead of another treatment?
- What exactly will the operation do?
- What will be removed during surgery?
- What are the chances of a cure?
- If I decide not to have surgery, what treatment will you recommend?
- Are there other possible treatments?
- What are the risks?
- What benefits will I receive from surgery that will outweigh the risks?
- What is your objective with the surgery?

- How long can I realistically postpone the surgery?
- What are the consequences if I decide not to have surgery?
- How long will I be in the hospital?
- When I awake after surgery, will I have any machines and tubes attached to me? What will they be? Why?
- How long will I have to stay at home recuperating?
- How long will it be before I am walking?
- How long will I miss work?
- How much pain will I experience? Where?
- What should I expect as after-effects?
- What do I have to do to prepare for the operation?
- Will I need assistance when I get home?
- What will it cost?

Radiation and chemotherapy treatments are similar in that both are typically administered through multiple sessions over a period of time. (See Chapter 8, Treatment.) Questions would include:

- What actually happens during the course of treatment?
- Why did you recommend this type of treatment?
- Why am I having this treatment instead of (or with) other treatments?
- What results do you expect to achieve with this treatment?
- Where will I get my treatments?
- Do I have a choice of facilities where I get treatments?
- Can I continue to work during the treatment period?

- How will I feel immediately after my treatment? How will I feel the day after treatment? How will I feel several days after treatment?
- How long will each treatment take?
- How often do I take a treatment?
- How many treatments will I have?
- What side effects can I expect?
- What are the risks?
- What will happen if I decide not to take this treatment?
- If I postpone this treatment, what are my risks?
- How long can I realistically wait to start treatment?
- How will you know if the treatment is doing any good?
- Can I take showers or baths after treatment?
- Will I be incapacitated? If "yes," for how long?
- After a treatment, when will I be able to go back to work?
- Will treatments affect my ability to drive an automobile?
- Will I experience sickness or pain?
- What precautions should I take before treatment?
- Will I be able to drink alcohol?
- Will I get depressed?
- What diet should I follow before and during the treatment period?
- Can I continue to take my regular medication?
- Who should I call if I have questions?
- After treatment, are there any symptoms that I should ignore?
- After treatment, are there typical "danger symptoms"

that might force me to contact you?
- Will I need help at home?
- If "yes," for how long?
- How much will my treatment cost?

The preceding questions will also apply to patients undergoing biological therapy. (See Chapter 8, Treatment.) Additional questions include:

- Is this treatment considered experimental?
- What is the history of this treatment? Where has it been tested? By what organization(s)?
- Why are you recommending a newer treatment instead of the more traditional treatments?

12

Is a Second Opinion Necessary?
THE PATIENT THINKING ONLY
ABOUT THE PATIENT

It is possible that the patient, at some point in the diagnosis process, will feel more secure by obtaining a second opinion. By all means, the patient should do so. Diagnosis is used to formulate and document a historical and current record of the illness. It does not normally cause any irreversible actions. In addition, diagnostic procedures such as the colonoscopy and barium enema can be repeated without causing the patient noticeable risk or pain.

When it comes to treatment, it is highly desirable to have a second opinion. Surgery cannot be reversed. Because all colorectal-cancer treatments are designed to impact the body in some way, no one should endure any treatments—surgery, radiation, chemotherapy or biological therapy—unless there are absolutely no other alternatives.

The idea behind the second opinion is not failure to trust a doctor. If trust and confidence are true considerations, the patient should skip second opinions and search for a new primary doctor. In fact, if the doctor is offended or if the response to the patient's request for a second opinion is negative in any way, the patient should consider finding another doctor.

Contrary to protests and denials from the medical profession, I have seen that some doctors do not appreciate second opinions. Some also seem to view answering a patient's probing questions as an imposition on their time. Fortunately, the vast majority of doctors enthusiastically encourage second opinions and questions, especially when the patient is confronting a serious illness such as cancer.

Five factors should lead a patient to securing a second opinion before surgery or any other cancer treatment is started:

1. The patient is the person who is about to endure a difficult experience. She or he should have an unlimited opportunity to learn and understand every aspect of what is about to occur. The patient is not exposed to added risk when obtaining a second opinion. Selecting the treatment could be the most important decision in the patient's life.
2. No doctor knows everything about everything. Nor is any doctor in the world mistake-free.
3. Cancer diagnosis and treatment are immense, complex medical fields. It is possible to reach different interpretations of the same set of facts and different solutions to the same problem.

4. Cancer study and research are producing a never-ending series of new theories, concepts, claims and methods. It is possible that a doctor has missed some relevant new development.

5. With the burdens and tensions of medical practice, it's conceivable a doctor, who might be treating another 200 patients, could overlook something during the diagnosis phase.

Getting a second opinion that contradicts the primary doctor's recommendation is not always a negative situation. It is better to hesitate if there is confusion than to proceed with an irreversible action. A better, faster, easier treatment may exist. With cancer, time is rarely of such essence that postponing treatment for a short time should not be a consideration.

The patient's responsibilities are to be forthright and honest with the primary doctor. He or she is a partner. The primary doctor should be told of the desire to get a second opinion, if for no other reason than he or she has the patient's records. These records could play a necessary and pivotal role in the second doctor's opinion. Further, doctors dealing with the same patient must have the opportunity to consult with one another. Very often, the primary doctor will be able to recommend a "second-opinion" doctor.

13

Searching for
Doctors & Hospitals
SATISFACTION WITH MEDICAL CARE

Internists are medical specialists who deal with innumerable inside-the-body organs and functions. Under the primary specialty of **Internal Medicine** are two subspecialities relating to colorectal-cancer patients.

Oncology is concerned with the study, diagnosis and treatment of tumors. It is essentially the field of medicine dealing with cancer. A doctor in this specialty is an oncologist.

Gastroenterology is the study, diagnosis and treatment of diseases and disorders found in the digestive system. A doctor in this specialty is a gastroenterologist.

Colon and Rectal Surgery is a primary specialty like Internal Medicine. Although there are surgeons who focus on cancer treatment, there is no recognized oncology surgery specialty. In most cases an oncologist, gastroenterologist or other doctor must make a recommendation before a surgeon will meet the patient.

Endoscopy is another descriptive medical term that can play a role in the diagnosis and treatment of colorectal cancer and polyps. This is an examination of the interior of the body. The *colonoscopy* and *sigmoidoscopy* are types of endoscopy examinations.

Proctology is a medical specialization dealing with the colon, rectum and anus. However, due to rapid changes in the fields of oncology and gastroenterology, the importance of proctology as a specialty is declining.

Colorectal cancer is a serious and complex condition, so diagnosis is best handled by a highly experienced specialist, such as a gastroenterologist or oncologist. In fact, when cancer is confirmed during the diagnosis phase, it is sometimes the best course of action to have treatment strategies handled by an oncologist. However, because oncology is a relatively new medical specialty, many older and experienced cancer doctors are not oncologists.

It is important to find the right specialist and/or to get a second opinion during the diagnosis period—before treatment begins. Several sources of information are available to the patient seeking either primary or second-opinion doctors.

1. In most cases a general practitioner, family doctor or internist is the first person to be in contact with the patient. This is often due to newly discovered

colorectal-cancer danger signs that appear as a result of symptoms or routine screening procedures. This first doctor should provide the referral to a specialist who will guide the patient through diagnosis and treatment. If the first referral proves to be unsatisfactory or if the patient needs a second opinion, there is no reason to hesitate in asking for another referral.

2. Although the National Cancer Institute (1-800-4-CANCER) and the American Cancer Society (1-800 ACS-2345) do not recommend specific doctors, both organizations will refer the caller to local medical referral sources. The local sources will, in turn, provide specific names, addresses and telephone numbers for nearby oncologists, gastroenterologists and other specialists.

3. Medical facilities participating in the National Cancer Institute's Community Oncology Program and/or the Cancer Center's Program are excellent sources for cancer research, diagnosis and treatment specialists. Refer to Appendixes E and F for information.

4. Hospitals with approved American College of Surgeons oncology programs have developed a credibility and reputation for cancer treatment. Twice a year the College of Surgeons publishes an extensive state-by-state list of hospitals with

approved oncology programs. To receive a free copy
of this booklet contact:

Commission on Cancer
Cancer Department
American College of Surgeons
55 East Erie Street
Chicago, IL 60611
(312) 664-4050

5. Many medical schools operate outpatient clinics that
will arrange appointments for cancer patients.

6. Many major hospitals have doctor-referral services.

7. Most public libraries have copies of the *Directory of
Medical Specialists* and/or the *American Medical
Directory*. These may be helpful in finding the names
of specialists and also in checking a doctor's credentials. The former is preferred because it deals only
with specialists. *The American Medical Directory* has a
much more general list, including all doctors who
are members of the American Medical Association.
In the *Directory of Medical Specialists* the colorectal-
cancer patient should look under "Internal
Medicine" for the subspecialties "Gastroenterology"
and "Medical Oncology." Also refer to the main specialty, "Colon and Rectal Surgery."

The Directory of Medical Specialists is organized by specialty, by state, by city, and by doctor in alphabetical order. The book's foreword explains the easy-to-understand codes used to describe a doctor's background. Information on individual doctors includes their age, medical schools, year licensed, primary and secondary specialties, type of practice, board certifications and hospital affiliations.

Specialty boards are private, independent organizations that establish qualifications and standards, as well as providing continuous education. Only after completing all training and residency requirements of a specialty can a doctor become eligible for certification. The certification itself is an involved process that includes rigorous written tests and oral examinations before other doctors who practice the specialty.

The American Board of Internal Medicine (1-800-441-2246) is the organization that handles certification for oncologists and gastroenterologists. The American Board of Surgery (1-215-568-4000) certifies surgeons. Most surgeons are also members of the American College of Surgeons. Further specialization comes with certification by the American Board of Colon and Rectal Surgery. The initials F.A.C.S. following a doctor's name indicate that he or she is a Fellow of the American College of Surgeons, a professional organization.

The American Board of Medical Specialties (ABMS) will supply certification information about any individual doctor. Its phone number is 1-800-776-CERT.

Board certification provides a strong indication that a doctor is well-trained and has proved a level of expertise to other doctors in the specialty. Certification is important because any licensed doctor, without any additional or special training, can legally call himself or herself anything from internist to surgeon.

However, even though board certification indicates a high level of competence, not all good specialists invest the time and effort necessary to get certified. They may spend their time and energy concentrating on research or teaching, so certification is not a consideration. And, as mentioned previously, oncology is a relatively new specialization. Some older, experienced cancer doctors are not board-certified. In fact, about one-fourth of the 600,000 practicing doctors in the U.S. do not have AMBS-recognized certification.

Another important aspect of a doctor's credentials is the quality of hospital affiliation. Any colorectal-cancer patient facing the prospect of an operation and hospital confinement must consider the quality of medical facilities of crucial importance. When evaluating a hospital, use the following criteria as guidelines:

1. Facilities affiliated with the National Cancer Institute and hospitals offering American College of Surgeons approved oncology programs are the best choices for a colorectal-cancer patient. (See Appendix E.)

2. About 500 hospitals are affiliated with medical schools. These hospitals attract top doctors to the faculty. They are usually well-staffed, offer a broad range of services and utilize state-of-the-art equipment.

3. Another 1500 hospitals have residency or internship programs although they are not affiliated with a medical school. They often offer more than hospitals without such programs.

4. Of the 7,000 hospitals in the United States, about 5,500 are accredited by the Joint Commission on Accreditation for Hospitals.

5. Private hospitals are often burdened with the pressures of producing a profit. In some instances, they do not have the latest equipment, lack internal controls and fail to offer the wide range of services found in other hospitals.

6. The size of the hospital can be indicative of the range of services and quality of facilities. The best-rated hospitals usually have over 500 beds. Those with fewer than 100 beds most often fall into the lowest ranking.

For the colorectal-cancer patient facing a possible operation, general hospital services should include:
- Postoperative recovery room
- Intensive Care Unit (ICU)
- Pathology laboratory
- Diagnostic laboratories
- Pharmacy
- Blood bank

- Current model X-ray equipment
- Diversified scanning equipment
- Physical therapy
- Social services
- Physician staffing 24 hours a day

8. *Anesthesiologists* are doctors whose specialty is the administering of anesthesia. *Anesthetists* are not doctors—they are usually trained nurses who give anesthesia under the direction of a doctor. The department of anesthesiology should be responsible for making sure an anesthesiologist is an integral member of every surgical team.

In the final analysis, the colorectal-cancer patient is putting his or her life into the hands of a doctor. In such circumstances, the importance of a patient's decisions when it comes to selecting a doctor cannot be overemphasized.

Section II

Prevention: The Impact of Diet

14

Polyp Prevention Trial

The medical community has concluded that most colorectal cancer evolves from adenomatous polyps, or adenomas. For the largest segment of society, i.e., those in the average-risk category, it is generally accepted that polyps develop, at least partially, as a result of poor diets. There are still many unanswered questions about polyps, but there is one indisputable fact: People who get polyps once are susceptible to getting them again. The National Cancer Institute estimates that almost half of all patients who have polyps removed will develop new ones.

Today, I am a participant in an extensive eight-year study that is attempting to prove the role of diet in causing polyps. The formal name for this jolly polyp brigade is the *Polyp Prevention Trial*. We go by PPT for short. I even have a big canvas shopping bag with *Polyp Prevention Trial* boldly embossed on the side. It was awarded to me as a bag of honor when the interviewing process was complete, and I was formally accepted for membership in this highly select group of polyp people. I carry it with pride.

Participation in the PPT is limited to people at least 35 years old who had at least one adenomatous polyp removed in the six-month period prior to joining the group. The premise of the PPT is to use a group of people who are likely to get the illness to test theories involving causes and cures. Although it is an eight-year study, each individual commits to a four-year period of involvement. The National Cancer Institute hopes to publish the results of the study sometime in 1998.

The PPT program is designed to show whether a low-fat/high-fiber diet will help prevent polyp recurrence. If this is shown to be the case among a group of high-risk people, the medical conclusion will be that similar eating habits will serve as an effective guard against developing polyps and colorectal cancer in the first place.

PPT Structure

The Polyp Prevention Trial is comprised of about 2,000 people split into two equal teams—the "Usual Diet Group" and the "Intervention Group."

Members of the Usual Diet Group are going about their lives in the same way as before, following their regular prior-to-polyps diets. The Intervention Group has gone through an orientation designed to modify their eating habits and are counseled regularly by trained nutritionists. These nutritionists instruct and encourage the participants in adopting an eating plan that is low in fat and high in fiber. I am a member of the Intervention Group.

Participants in both groups return to their doctors for regular checkups. Whenever more polyps are discovered in members of either group, the polyps are removed. After completion of the program, the polyp frequencies of the two groups will be compared to reach conclusions about the role of diet in preventing polyps.

The PPT is no fly-by-night study group. It is a federally funded project conducted by the National Cancer Institute (NCI) of the National Institutes of Health (NIH). The entire effort is coordinated through the NCI national headquarters in the Washington, D.C. area. Medical professionals at seven major facilities are involved in the program:

- Edward Hines VA Hospital, Illinois
- Kaiser Foundation Research Institute, California
- Memorial-Sloan Kettering Cancer Center, New York
- University of Buffalo, New York
- University of Pittsburgh, Pennsylvania
- University of Utah, Utah
- Wake Forest University, North Carolina
- Walter Reed Army Medical Center, Washington, DC

The 1,000 members of the Intervention Group were required to sign formal releases and to commit to following a nonbreakable lowfat, high-fiber diet that includes lots of fruits and vegetables. We also had to agree to meet for counseling sessions with a PPT nutritionist, according to the following schedule:

Year 1	Weekly—for 6 sessions, then
	Biweekly—for 3 sessions, then
	Monthly—for 9 sessions
Year 2	Bimonthly—6 sessions
Years 3-4	Quarterly—8 sessions

To get an idea of the size of this effort, consider the manpower involved in getting me through the first three months of the program. I had a two-hour orientation followed by the nine counseling sessions for a total of 11 hours of one-to-one nutritional counseling. The 1,000 members of the Intervention Group required 11,000 hours of PPT professional staff manpower—just to get through the beginning phases of the program! This figure does not include the work of the Washington-based management and administrative personnel, nor that of the on-site clinical centers' support staffs. It also does not include the orientation requirements for the Usual Diet Group. Most remarkable is the fact that the beginning 11,000 hours of manpower investment only serves to get everyone started. Almost another four years of PPT teaching and monitoring work remains to be accomplished.

It will cost the government over $25 million to develop and complete the lowfat/high-fiber PPT project. Why go to this expense? Quite probably, it is the startling statistics concerning colorectal cancer that provide the motivation: Each year, more than a million Americans are diagnosed with polyps and 150,000 Americans are diagnosed with colorectal cancer. About 50,000 deaths annually are directly attributable to colorectal cancer—one-half million deaths during every decade. Considering the risks and human suffering, the investment in dollars seems insignificant.

PPT Computer-Generated Diet Assessment

As part of the PPT interviewing process, each participant completed a detailed Food Questionnaire concerning past eating habits. These were evaluated by computer. My computer-generated eating analysis appears on the following page.

    PPT diet goals are:

- 20% of calories from fat
- 18 grams of fiber per 1,000 calories
- 5 to 8 servings per day of fruits and vegetables, depending on total caloric intake.

Based on my Food Questionaire, the computer estimated my average caloric consumption at 2,218 calories a day. In the past this included 105 grams of fat, 12 grams of fiber and 2.2 servings of fruits and vegetables. My weight fluctuated between 205 and 215 pounds, acceptable for my 6-foot frame. My PPT daily consumption goals were set at 49 grams of fat, 40 grams of fiber and 8 servings of fruits and vegetables. For the PPT, caloric intake is inconsequential. Yet, by lowering my fat intake and consuming more high-fiber foods, fruits and vegetables, I reduced my daily calories by 15% to 30%.

    The computer-generated program provides a great amount of useful information concerning past eating habits and future goals. In the lower right are my old levels (baseline) and new PPT goals for fat, fiber and fruit/vegetables.

POLYP PREVENTION TRIAL SUMMARY SHEET
Food Frequency Analysis
Date 12/11/92

Participant ID: 60741   Nutritionist: L. Cohen
Visit Code: TO   Nutritionist ID: 35

	Your Average Daily Intake	% of Total Calories	Recommended % of Total Calories
Calories	2217.9		
Protein (g)	98.0	17.7	10%-15%
Carbohydrates (g)	196.8	35.5	55%-65%
Fat (g)	104.9	42.6	30% (max.)
Fiber (g/1000 calories)	5.3	N/A	
Alcohol (calories)	107.7	4.9	

Vitamins, Minerals & Fiber	Your Average Daily Intake			
	Food	Supplements	Total	RDAs*
Vitamin A (RE)	667.2	571.6	1238.8	800-1000 RE
Vitamin C (mg)	47.4	57.2	104.6	60-100 mg
Thiamine-B1 (mg)	1.2	6.0	7.2	1.0-1.5 mg
Riiboflavin-B2 (mg)	1.4	6.8	8.2	1.2-1.7 mg
Niacin-B3 (mg)	27.0	60.0	87.0	13-19 mg
Calcium, (mg)	573.3	0.0	573.3	800-1200 mg
Sodium (mg)	2982.1	N/A	2982.1	*Recommended Daily
Fiber (g)	11.7	0.0	11.7	Allowances. National Academy of Sciences

Weekly Frequency of Selected Foods

	servings
Fruit	3.8
Fruit Juice	0.5
Vegetable	11.5
Whole-Grain Bread/Starch	1.8
Fiber Cereals	0.0
Fish/Chicken	6.8
Beef/Pork	2.8
Breakfast Meats	0.0
Hot Dogs/Lunch Meat	0.3
Eggs	3.3
Butter/Margarine	6.5
Milk/Yogurt	0.5
Cheese (excl. cottage/lowfat)	3.3
Frozen Dessert	0.3
Other Desserts	3.3
Alcohol	6.2

	Fat grams	Fiber grams	F&V servings
Baseline	104.9	11.7	2.2
	(intake before PPT)		
Goal	49.3	39.9	8.0
	(goals set by PPT computer)		

Polyp Prevention Trial
Guide To Dietary Intake Assessment
(Information provided to all PPT participants)

This dietary assessment [shown on previous page] describes your intake of calories, protein, carbohydrates, fat and fiber, as well as some of the major vitamins and minerals. Your nutrient intake is reported as an average value determined from your responses to the Food Questionnaire.

Your nutrient intakes from foods and from vitamin and mineral supplements are listed in separate columns. For many of these nutrients we included a recommended range to meet the needs of most healthy persons. Most values are the Recommended Dietary Allowances (RDAs) established by the National Research Council. They should not be confused with individual requirements, which may vary considerably according to age, body size, state of health and lifestyle.

Here is a description of the functions of the major nutrients and a listing of the primary food sources.

Calories are derived from the protein, fats and carbohydrates in food and from alcohol. We all need calories for daily living, but the amount varies for each person depending on age, sex, height, weight and physical activity.

Protein is an essential component making up your body's cells. Approximately 12% to 15% of your total calories should come from protein. Excess protein will be stored as fat in the body, as will an excess of fat or carbohydrate.

Sources: meat, poultry, fish, milk, cheese, eggs, dried beans and peas

Fats supply a large amount of energy in a small amount of food, providing twice as many calories per ounce as carbohydrates and proteins. Fats are also utilized in the production of body cells and hormones.

Sources: fatty meats, sausage, bacon, cream, cheese, butter, whole milk, oil, margarine and salad dressings

Carbohydrates are the major sources of energy both for the body's internal functioning and for physical activity. They also help maintain body temperature. 55% to 60% of your total calories should come from carbohydrates, primarily complex sources.

There are two types of carbohydrates: simple and complex. Simple carbohydrates are sugars such as sucrose (table sugar), which provide calories but little else in the way of nutrients.

Complex carbohydrates are starches and dietary fiber. Most foods high in complex carbohydrates supply vitamins and minerals. Dietary fiber, which is part of the nondigestible component of carbohydrates, provides bulk in the diet and aids in elimination and in the prevention of bowel problems. Scientific organizations suggest a minimum of 20 grams of fiber daily. It is advised that we increase our intake of foods through fiber-rich foods and not supplements.

Sources: *Simple carbohydrates*—all sugars, syrups, honey, candy, regular soft drinks, cakes and cookies

Sources: *Complex carbohydrates*—whole-grains (wheat, rye, oat, corn, barley), whole-grain breads and cereals, fruits, vegetables, beans and peas

VITAMINS AND MINERALS

Vitamin A occurs in two major forms: retinol, found in animal sources, and carotene, found in vegetable sources. This vitamin is important for normal mucous membranes, good vision, normal bone growth and healthy skin and hair.

Sources: *Retinol*—liver and fish liver oils; egg yolk, red meats, butter and margarine also have small amounts

Sources: *Carotene*—carrots, broccoli, deep-green and leafy vegetables, cantaloupe and apricots

Vitamin C (ascorbic acid) is essential for maintaining healthy teeth, gums and bones, for building strong cells and blood vessels, for healing wounds and broken bones, and for resisting infections.

Sources: citrus fruits, strawberries, broccoli and tomatoes

B Vitamins include thiamine, riboflavin and niacin. All are essential for protein, fat and energy metabolism. They are important for the maintenance of healthy blood vessels and cells, teeth and gums, and a healthy nervous and cardiovascular system.

Sources: whole grains, eggs, vegetables, fish and poultry

Calcium: A low calcium intake is one of the dietary factors associated with *osteoporosis*, a disease characterized by a decrease in the amount of bone, which can lead to easy fractures.

Sources: dairy products—milk, yogurt, cheese, ice cream and dark-green vegetables

Sodium: Table salt, made from sodium and chloride, provides most of the sodium in our diets. Most Americans consume more salt and sodium than they need. High blood pressure is less common in populations with diets low in salt. A diet with less salt may help some people reduce their risk of developing high blood pressure.

Sources: salt, salted chips, crackers, pretzels, nuts, pickles, olives, some processed meats and cheeses, and many frozen meals and fast foods

---

Computer Calculation of PPT Fat Goal

2218	daily caloric intake
20%	PPT goal of 20% calories from fat. This equals:
444	calories from fat
÷ 9	number of grams of fat in each calorie
49	grams of fat a day, the PPT goal

Computer Calculation of PPT Fiber Goal

2218	daily caloric intake goal
÷1000	
2.2	units of 1,000 calories per day
x 18	grams of fiber per 1,000 calories.
40	grams of fiber a day, the PPT goal

Authorities such as the American Cancer Society recommend that daily maximum fiber intake should be 35 grams. The PPT explanation for my higher goal is that the PPT eating plan emphasizes *high* fiber consumption. I am keeping my goal at 40 grams a day. My current level of fiber intake ranges from 30 to 40 grams a day.

On the other hand, the American Cancer Society has determined that a person requires only about 25 grams of fat a day. Although the PPT set my goal at 49 grams, I cut my daily fat intake to 20 to 30 grams. An unexpected result of the decrease in fat consumption was a decrease of my total calories to 1600 to 1800 per day—down from 2,218.

After about three months, my eating habits changed radically. The PPT graphs that monitored consumption of fat and fiber show these changes.

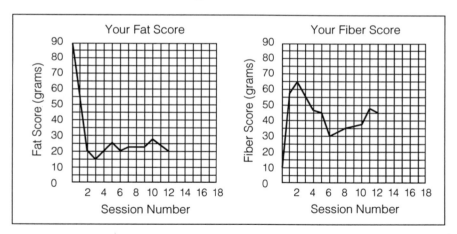

My reactions to the PPT are not unique. The following performance graphs show the average changes in the eating habits of all 1000 members of the PPT Intervention Group after about one year into the four-year program.

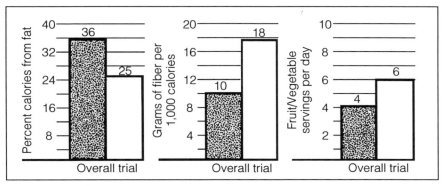

PPT PERFORMANCE ANALYSIS
Shaded areas represent average consumption for participants before PPT. White areas represent participants' average consumption about a year after they started the PPT program.

The Non-Diet Diet

The PPT is a two-part program: First, it supplies education about the foods we eat. Second, it provides a training program to help us develop good eating habits.

The educational phase includes a review of the diet material (*not* the medical information) included in this book. It is a general introduction to the benefits of healthy eating and emphasizes the importance of a diet low in fat, high in fiber and including lots of fruits and vegetables.

Every friend and business associate over 40 years of age who knows of my illness and participation in the PPT has asked in vain for a copy of my new diet. There is none. The objective of the PPT is not to give us a quick-fix diet that will last for a few weeks or months but to help us develop an eating discipline to carry through the rest of our lives. Just as the immigrant disembarking from a ship in New York harbor has to learn how to communicate in a new and unfamiliar language, I am learning new and unfamiliar ways to eat.

The underlying purpose of PPT training is a subtle form of mind control. The PPT truly is a "head game." It is a psychological challenge to change eating habits that have been a part of my life for over 50 years. Understand this retraining is a day-in/day-out endeavor brimming with constant temptation. Everybody tells me I'm going to learn to *like* vegetables and fruit. And soon I will not miss my rare steaks and baked potatoes drenched in butter sauce. Bull! I don't believe it. Rest assured, I will never enjoy a bowl of spinach as much as I enjoy veal parmigiana.

The 20/20 Lists

Soon after joining the PPT, I prepared my own lists of 20 high-fat foods to avoid and 20 high-fiber foods to include in my diet. Neatly written on index cards, my 20/20 lists form the basis of my new eating discipline. I avoid the foods on list #1 and gradually add those on list #2. I concentrate on foods I like and add in plenty of my favorite fruits and vegetables.

These lists are my key reference tools. They have been invaluable in helping me achieve my daily goals of no more than 25 grams of fat and 40 grams of fiber.

#1 HIGH-FAT FOODS TO AVOID

1. Meats, bacon, sausages, cold cuts
2. Cheeses
3. Whole milk, cream, half-and-half
4. Sour cream
5. Cottage cheese, cream cheese
6. Mayonnaise
7. Butter, margarine
8. Cream soups
9. Vegetable oils
10. Pies, cakes
11. White bread, croissants, doughnuts
12. Eggs
13. Chocolate, candy, ice cream
14. Pizza
15. Olives
16. Nuts, seeds, coconut
17. Peanut butter
18. French fries, onion rings
19. Avocado
20. Fast-food restaurants

#2 HIGH-FIBER FOODS TO EAT

1. Chicken, turkey
2. Fish
3. Whole-grain breads
4. Wild rice
5. High-fiber cereals & raisin bran
6. Oatmeal
7. Beans, beans, beans
8. Raspberries, strawberries
9. Apples, pears, unpeeled
10. Figs, apricots, prunes
11. Corn, broccoli, Brussels sprouts
12. Baked potatoes, unpeeled
13. Chili (no meat)
14. Vegetable lasagna
15. Sauerkraut, sweet potatoes
16. Artichokes, asparagus, carrots
17. Raisins, bananas
18. Whole-wheat pasta
19. Steamed Chinese food & brown rice
20. Barley & bean soup

15

Getting Rid of the Fat

The first objective for the PPT Intervention Group is to get rid of most of the fat in our diets. A high-fat diet is the connection that links heart disease and bowel cancer. Somewhere at the center of any discussion dealing with the causes of these two deadly diseases is consumption of fat in the human diet.

Fat, protein and carbohydrates all provide energy in the form of calories, but fat has more than twice as many calories as the other two—nine calories per gram of fat compared to four calories per gram of carbohydrates or protein. Reduce the amount of fat in your diet and you will automatically achieve a dramatic reduction in calories.

Just as there is no longer any debate about smoking being the primary cause of lung cancer, this world has come to understand that high-fat diets are also potentially dangerous. It is now considered a medical fact that if you eat too much fat you dramatically increase the risks of developing a number of serious illnesses, ranging from colorectal cancer to heart disease.

Although our bodies require some fat to accomplish an assortment of life-support functions, most of us eat far more than we need. In the typical American diet, fat accounts for about 40% of the day's calories. A general rule of thumb is that an adult should get no more than 20% of caloric intake from fat.

A serving of food is usually measured in ounces. The amount of fat in food is usually measured in grams. One ounce of anything is equal to 28 grams. A paper clip weighs about one gram, a penny about three grams.

Each gram of fat contains 9 calories, so to find out how many grams of fat will provide the 20% allowed you, divide the allowable fat calories by 9. In the following chart, for example, a woman whose recommended diet contains 1500 calories should get no more than 300 calories from fat. This is equivalent to 33 grams of fat. A man who eats 2500 calories per day would be allowed 500 calories, or 56 grams of fat. There are those who claim that any healthy person actually needs far less than that—about 10 to 20 grams of fat a day.

Obtaining 20% of Calories from Fat

Formula Example:

Daily Calories	1500
x 20% Calories from Fat	x .20
Total Calories from Fat	300
Divided by Grams of Fat in Each Calorie	÷ 9
Daily Consumption of Fat Grams	33

20% of Calories from Fat

Daily Calorie Consumption	Total Calories From Fat	Grams of Fat
1300	260	29
1500	300	33
1700	340	38
1900	380	42
2100	420	47
2300	460	51
2500	500	56
2700	540	60
2900	580	64

Before I changed my eating habits, my average daily consumption of fat exceeded 100 grams. Today, it is less than 30 grams. My new eating habit has become a discipline—one that was born out of fear and nurtured with knowledge. I still enjoy eating a small piece of chocolate, but butter, sour cream and red meats have been eliminated or replaced with lowfat or no-fat substitutes.

Surprisingly, the most difficult task is being aware of what is in the food I eat. The act of eating correctly has now become a comfortable and unconscious way of life. For information on the fat content of specific foods, refer to the food tables in Appendix A.

There are two main classifications of fats. *Saturated fats* remain solid at room temperature. They are generally found in animal products such as meat, and dairy products such as butter, cream, whole milk and ice cream. Several vegetable products, including tropical oils such as coconut and palm oil, and cocoa butter (used in making chocolate), are also high in saturated fats. Saturated fats are considered the most dangerous and should be avoided.

Unsaturated fats are characterized by being liquid at room temperature. There are two categories of unsaturated fat. *Polyunsaturated* fats are liquid at room temperature and also when cold. Polyunsaturated fats are comprised mainly of plant and vegetable oils such as corn, cottonseed, sunflower and soybean oil. *Monounsaturated fats* are liquid at room temperature but change into a more solid form when cold. Monounsaturated fats are the *least harmful* and include olive oil, peanut oil, sesame oil and canola oil.

Foods made with liquid fats do not have as long a shelf life as those made with solid fats. Food-processing companies employ a chemical process called *hydrogenation* to transform liquid fats into solids, called *trans fats*. Unfortunately, this makes them more like saturated fats. For the informed shopper, the word *hydrogenation* on a label for foods such as margarines and cookies is a warning that the chemically produced and harmful trans fats are present.

All types of fat are difficult for the body to digest. In addition, no food has only one type of fat content. For example, avocados are rich in monounsaturated fat, but also contain a lot of saturated fat. It is important to be aware of the type of fat you are eating because some types are more harmful than others.

The most important fact a survivor needs to keep in mind is that *fat is a killer*. One factor contributing to heart disease is bad eating habits that include foods having high levels of fat. It is also widely accepted that high-fat diets are a factor in digestive disorders ranging from polyps to colorectal cancer. Fat is a substance that causes pain, disease and death.

With the information available today, it is inconceivable anyone could argue that fat in food is harmless. The fact is, the adage, "Eating what you like is one of life's greatest pleasures," describes a game of Russian roulette when it comes to consuming fat.

Suggestions for Cutting Down Fat Intake

- Keep meat consumption down to once or twice a week. Eat smaller portions. Avoid red meat, which is high in saturated fat. Choose lean cuts and trim away all noticeable fat before cooking. Avoid processed meats such as bacon, sausage, hot dogs, cold cuts and all fat-marbled meats. Lean cuts of beef and veal have less fat than lamb and pork.
- Eat more poultry such as chicken and turkey. Turkey has less fat than chicken. White meat has less fat than dark meat. Small birds have less fat than larger ones. Use two small chickens instead of a large one. Remove all visible fat before cooking.
- Fish is generally low in fat. Fish with higher fat content includes salmon, tuna, mackerel, blue fish,

herring, anchovies, sardines, shad and trout. For canned fish such as tuna, choose water-packed rather than oil-packed brands.

•Choose cooking methods that add no fats to foods: bake, steam, poach, roast or use a microwave oven. If you must fry food, use a non-stick pan with a cooking spray instead of adding oil. Broil, bake or grill meats on a rack so the fat drips away during the cooking process.

•Add flavor to steamed vegetables without adding fat by cooking them over water mixed with herbs, vinegar, wine, fresh ginger, soy sauce, or combinations of these ingredients.

•Make a lowfat "cream" soup by adding 1/2 cup puréed white rice to a quart of soup. The puréed rice gives the soup the same "mouth feel" as fat does.

•Make a lowfat sauce by puréeing cooked vegetables with their cooking liquid. Add salt, thyme, sage, oregano, or other herbs and enough additional water to make the sauce the desired consistency.

•Be wary of foods labeled as containing "vegetable oil." This may mean coconut oil or palm oil, which are high in saturated fats.

•Substitute lowfat or fat-free cheese for cheeses with high fat content. Lowfat cheeses include alpine lace, Swiss lorraine and fat-free Cheddar. Use Parmesan, part-skim mozzarella and part-skim ricotta in moderation.

- Substitute plain lowfat or no-fat yogurt or lowfat or no-fat cottage cheese for sour cream on baked potatoes or in making tuna and potato salads. Use fat-free or reduced-fat mayonnaise instead of regular mayonnaise.

- Choose lowfat or no-fat margarines instead of butter for spreads and cooking. Cut down on margarine and butter as a sauce for vegetables, rice and potatoes. Softer margarine usually contains less saturated fat. For example, tub margarine is better than stick margarine. In cooking, use safflower, walnut and sunflower oils instead of butter or margarine.

- Substitute skim (no-fat) or 1%-fat milk in recipes and for drinking. Use evaporated skim milk instead of cream in coffee and tea. Avoid half-and-half, cream and light cream, which are monster sources of fat.

- Use lowfat or no-fat salad dressings.

- Use dry cereals as snack foods, but beware of granola, which is naturally high in fat. Pretzels are good low-fat snacks, so is "light" microwave popcorn. The best low-fat snack is dry or fresh fruit.

- For desserts, try lowfat or no-fat frozen yogurts, or lowered-fat ice creams. An ever-increasing assortment of fat-free bakery goods is now available.

- Season foods with herbs and spices instead of margarine or butter. Lemon juice, mustard, salsa and picante sauce are lowfat seasonings and condiments.

- Toss grains and rice with citrus juice and/or zest of citrus fruits (finely grated peel) to enhance flavor without adding fat. Use grated zest as a flavorful alternative to butter or margarine in vegetable dishes.

• Make a lowfat garlic bread by spreading crusty Italian or French bread slices with roasted garlic. To roast garlic, bake whole (unpeeled) garlic heads at 375F (190C) in your oven or toaster oven for 30 to 45 minutes or until the heads feel soft when squeezed. Squeeze the roasted garlic out of head onto bread slices and spread.

• Avoid white bread, which may contain as much as 150 calories and 10 grams of fat per slice. Many types of dark, whole-grain breads are lower in fat. They are also quite flavorful and do not need as much (or any) spread. Instead of butter or margarine, use lowfat or no-fat spreads. Use lowfat or no-fat jams and jellies.

• Avoid fast-food restaurants.

• Avoid chocolate, avocados (a single medium avocado has 30.8 grams of fat) and all nuts. Fat content of nuts ranges from about 10 grams to 100 grams of fat per cup.

• Ketchup and mustard are fat-free. Use them rather than mayonnaise on sandwiches. Or perk up a sandwich with a mixture of fat-free mayonnaise, a spice such as chili powder, and a couple of drops of hot sauce.

• Make soups and stews the day before serving and refrigerate them overnight. The next day, skim off the fat, which will have risen and congealed on the surface.

•Read food labels carefully. The suggested serving size may be unrealistically low. Also "lowfat" is a relative term that often means the product is a lower-fat version of the original product. It still may contain more fat than you wish to eat.

The Cholesterol Connection

It is impossible to carry on a discussion about fats in food without mentioning *cholesterol*. An added benefit of a lowfat diet is lowering cholesterol.

Fat and cholesterol are not the same. Carbohydrates, protein and fat are nutrients. They provide calories that act as energy fuel for the body. Cholesterol is not a nutrient, but it is a vital body chemical. Among other functions, it is used to make cell membranes and it may aid in digestion.

There are two sources of cholesterol. One is cholesterol made by a built-in body manufacturing process. The other is the cholesterol from food of animal origin, the same source as saturated fats. Interestingly, an egg yolk, with over 250 milligrams of cholesterol, is one of the most concentrated sources of cholesterol in the American diet. Egg whites, however, are an excellent, cholesterol-free source of protein.

The body produces all the cholesterol it needs. So when food with cholesterol is eaten, the usual result is a cholesterol oversupply.

Whether it is from food or manufactured by the body, cholesterol is a waxlike substance that travels through the body via the bloodstream. Problems develop when too much cholesterol clogs up the arteries and interferes with the flow of blood.

Cholesterol is expressed as the amount of cholesterol, measured in milligrams, in a volume of blood, which is measured in deciliters. A cholesterol reading falls onto a scale used to define the cholesterol level in terms of cardiac risk. The higher the cholesterol level, the greater the risk.

The National Institutes of Health has established general guidelines as to cholesterol risk, as shown below.

It is hard to imagine anyone having a cholesterol level that is too low. The lower the better is the acceptable rule. Although safe levels for cholesterol are normally considered to be under 200, many doctors believe that risk actually begins when the cholesterol level passes 150. Some medical authorities recommend medical supervision when cholesterol levels surpass 240.

Cardiac Risk vs. Cholesterol and Age

Age	Moderate Risk (mg/dl)	High Risk (mg/dl)
20-29	200-220	greater than 220
30-39	220-240	greater than 240
40 and over	240-260	greater than 260

16

The Importance of Fiber

For years I've known that smoking is hazardous to my health. I may not know all the medical reasons, but after all the powerful publicity, I do not question the conclusions. I'm also convinced that a diet with too much fat is a primary reason for heart disease and colorectal cancer. Again, I do not fully understand why. But the never-ending flow of information from all sources trumpeting the self-destructive qualities of fat leads me to believe that fat is not good for me.

But *fiber* and my health? Before my illness, I didn't even know what or where fiber was, let alone why it was supposed to be good for me.

Fiber is what my mother called *roughage* or *bulk*. Fiber is a substance obtained from plants. It cannot be digested but passes through the digestive system from start to finish basically intact. It is a low-calorie way to fill the stomach and quench hunger.

Numerous kinds of fiber are found in an assortment of foods. The body needs a variety of fiber from different food sources. To limit fiber intake to a few foods or a fiber supplement is not recommended.

Fiber's role is to enhance the formation and movement of stools, a process that occurs in the large bowel. Proper intake of fiber will stimulate the smooth and efficient working of the large bowel. Fiber has a sponge-like quality that absorbs liquids and binds food waste together as it makes its way through the digestive system. People who eat too little fiber tend to produce stools that are hard, dry, small and difficult to pass out of the body. Fiber naturally leads to the creation of soft, bulky stools, so waste moves easily through the colon and rectum.

If a person has a constant need to exert pressure and must strain to pass stools, this will, in time, harm the digestive system. Irregularity and irritation are often traced to inadequate intake of fiber, which frequently is the source for colorectal disorders.

On the average, Americans eat about 8 to 12 grams of fiber a day. Most authorities recommend that Americans should double the amount of fiber they eat to 20 to 30 grams. The National Cancer Institute has suggested that daily intake should not exceed 65 grams. Not understanding the word *moderation* regarding any facet of my life, I started consuming over 70 grams of fiber soon after beginning a lowfat/high-fiber diet. Within a few days, I developed constant diarrhea, accompanied by embarrassing intestinal gas. I immediately cut back the fiber. Today, I am experiencing near-perfect regularity, once every morning.

As I learned the hard way, fiber should be added to a diet gradually, beginning with small portions of food containing fiber. If fiber is introduced too rapidly into one's diet, there is a danger of experiencing painful stomach cramps, excessive gas and diarrhea.

Along with the fiber, medical experts strongly recommend that a person drink 8 to 10 glasses of liquid a day. The PPT plan encourages this, making it a high-fiber/lowfat/lots-of-fruits-and-vegetables/much-liquid eating discipline!

Medical research and mounting circumstantial evidence support the theory that many digestive disorders can be traced back to improper diets that are prevalent in the industrialized societies of the western world. Today almost all doctors attest to the attributes of lowfat/high-fiber diets.

Certain irrefutable facts are enlightening:

• First fact: Throughout the world, one-half million people will be diagnosed with colorectal cancer every year. Millions of people will be diagnosed as having polyps.

• Second fact: Underdeveloped, third-world countries typically follow high-fiber/lowfat diets with substantial consumption of fruits and vegetables. Colorectal problems are rare in these countries.

• Third fact: In the industrialized societies of the western world, colorectal disorders are reaching epidemic proportions.

These introductory facts might be a result of factors other than an improper diet. Differences in lineage (i.e., race), locale or environment could be causes of colorectal cancer. However, further investigation eliminates such considerations.

- Fourth fact: People who have migrated from the underdeveloped regions to developed areas of the world are today as susceptible to bowel disorders as are "natives" of developed countries. For example, people of Japanese origin who moved to the United States in the 1940s and embraced the American way of life have as much risk of developing colorectal disorders as other Americans. Japanese living in Japan who follow traditional lowfat/high-fiber diets have relatively few colorectal problems.

- Fifth fact: There is an increase in the incidence of bowel cancer in countries that are developing or becoming westernized. For example, in major urban centers of Japan, bowel-cancer rates are now rising about 5% a year. In remote country villages, there has been no change.

- Sixth fact: Bowel cancer in a low-risk country is most common among its richer, urbanized members.

- Seventh Fact: In America, young adults usually pass food through the digestive system within 3 days. For the elderly, it could take more than a week.

Average stools normally weigh 3 to 5 ounces. In most parts of Africa and Asia, young adults pass food in 30 to 40 hours and stools weigh over a pound.

For the million-plus average-risk Americans who will develop colorectal cancer this decade, medical research has eliminated as possible causes many of the environmental elements and personal living habits known to cause other forms of cancer. Some new studies have indicated possible increased colorectal-cancer risks associated with long-term, heavy smoking. Personal hygiene, sexual activity, sunlight, climate and air pollution do not appear to have any bearing on the development of colorectal cancer and polyps.

Thus, little remains as a possible cause of colorectal cancer except diet. If you think of the digestive tract as a food-processing plant, it makes sense that what you put (or don't put) into the processor is the cause of the problem. When the lungs inhale smoke, lung cancer is often the result. When the digestive system consumes the wrong combinations of foods, the result can be colorectal cancer.

A 20-year-old medical study conducted by Denis Burkitt, an English doctor working in Africa, remains a primary and authoritative source for researchers dealing with the impact of fiber. In the early 1970s, Dr. Burkitt wrote that his African patients rarely suffered from bowel afflictions common in the industrialized world. He observed that American Whites and American Blacks were equally susceptible to colorectal disorders. Burkitt therefore quickly eliminated genetic background as a contributing reason for the near-absence of digestive problems in his African patients. After in-depth studying of normal diets, plus highly technical analysis of the excretion process and stool, he concluded that fiber was a primary differentiating factor between African diets and diets of the western world. Supported by his research results, Dr. Burkitt pinpointed consistent intake of high-fiber foods as a primary reason his African patients lacked digestive-tract problems. The indigestible aspect of fiber left little doubt as to its presence in the stools.

A 1987 National Cancer Institute release mirrored Dr. Burkitt's findings by stating, "Dietary fiber and its interaction with fat remains the single-most comprehensive explanation of the causation of bowel cancer."

A March 1992 article in the *Journal of the American Medical Association* underscores the importance of eating habits as they relate to digestive-tract disorders. In summarizing a study conducted by the Harvard School of Public Health, the *Journal* reported:*

> **Background:** Rates of colorectal cancer in various countries are strongly correlated with per capita consumption of red meat and animal fat and inversely associated with fiber consumption. There have been few studies, however, of dietary-risk factors for colorectal adenomas, which are precursors of cancer.

*E. Giovannucci, "Relationship of Diet to Risk of Colorectal Adenoma in Men." JAMA March 1992, p. 1595.

Purpose: Our purpose was to determine prospectively the relationship between dietary factors and risk of colorectal adenomas.

Conclusions: These prospective data provide evidence for the hypotheses that a diet high in saturated fat and low in fiber increases the risk for colorectal adenoma. They also support existing recommendations to substitute chicken and fish for red meat in the diet and to increase intake of vegetables, fruits and grains to reduce risk of colorectal cancer.

Unless prescribed by a doctor, medical experts suggest that fiber supplements should not be used as a substitute for dietary fiber from food sources. Such supplements do not have vitamins, minerals or other nutritional qualities found in food. Furthermore, the body needs a variety of fibers that can come only from an assortment of different foods. Reliance on the same types of fiber found in a particular supplement is not beneficial and could actually be harmful. Commercial fiber supplements are not laxatives, regardless of manufacturers' claims. Rather, supplements contain fiber, which enhances the movement of bowels.

Additionally, users of laxatives should be on guard. Although it is impossible to define normal bowel movement in terms of number during the day or time of day, it is not normal to miss moving one's bowels on any day. And, it is not normal to solve the problem by regular ingestion of laxatives. When overused, laxatives tend to create dependencies and can lead to a form of addiction. Dependence on laxatives can be as dangerous to one's health as a diet without sufficient fiber and liquids.

Suggestions For Increasing Consumption of High-Fiber Foods

•Legumes are rich in fiber, low in fat, a good protein source, low in sodium and a supplier of B vitamins, magnesium, iron and potassium. Legumes include baked beans, kidney beans, split peas, lima beans, garbanzos, pinto beans, black beans, red beans, green beans and lentils. In addition to being eaten alone, beans are perfectly suited to being mixed with salads and other vegetables. Also, a wide variety of flavorful bean and pea soups are available that possess the same excellent food qualities. Cook beans thoroughly—until they are soft and mash easily.

•Dried fruits, especially figs, apricots, prunes, raisins, dates, peaches and pears, are excellent sources of fiber.

•Raspberries, blackberries, strawberries and all kinds of berries, especially those filled with seeds, are good fiber sources.

•Whenever possible, do not peel fruits and vegetables before eating. Most of the fiber and nutrients are stored in and near the skin. Raw fruits and vegetables have more fiber than when cooked.

• Broccoli and Brussels sprouts are primary fiber vegetables.

• Baked potatoes (with the skins) are good fiber sources.

• Use quick-cooking barley or bulgur instead of white rice or noodles in casseroles, stews, soups, side dishes and salads.

• Try cooked bulgur as a hot breakfast cereal, substituting apple juice for half the cooking liquid and adding dried or fresh fruit.

• Substitute bulgur or quick-cooking barley for some of the ground meat in chili, tacos, stuffed peppers, hamburgers and meat loaf.

• Toss fresh or thawed frozen vegetables, such as broccoli, cauliflower, carrots or peas, into green or pasta salads.

• Create new salads based on corn, beans, broccoli, peas, winter squash and other vegetables, alone or in combination.

• Add fresh, frozen or canned vegetables to your favorite soups.

•Add orange segments, dried fruit or chopped pears and apples to chicken, tuna and green salads.

•Look for ways to include dried and fresh fruit in main dishes. They are especially good with chicken and curry dishes.

•Top lowfat or fat-free frozen yogurt with fresh or frozen berries.

•Nuts, especially almonds, Brazil nuts, peanuts, walnuts, cashews, pinenuts, pecans and pistachio nuts, are high-fiber sources, as are coconuts. But consume nuts sparingly because of their high fat content.

•Contrary to food-manufacturers' claims, not all grain products are high in fiber. A clue to a food's fiber content is whether it is made from *whole grains*. Examples of whole grains include whole wheat, bulgur, oatmeal, popcorn, brown rice, whole rye and scotch barley. Processing removes fiber, vitamins and minerals from the rich, whole grains. Because of this, it is a good idea to avoid white flour, white rice and most types of cornmeal. Be on guard for foods claiming to be *enriched*. This is often just another word for *processed*. A common example is enriched white bread.

•Cereals are not always what they appear to be. Be particularly careful when selecting granola cereals; most are very high in fat. Whole-grain and bran cereals are good fiber sources. Most special high-fiber cereals such as Kellogg's All-Bran with Extra Fiber® and General Mills Fiber One® have more than 10 grams of fiber per 1/2-cup serving. If a breakfast consisting exclusively of high-fiber cereals does not sound appetizing, try mixing together equal parts of raisin bran and a high-fiber cereal. For taste and more fiber, add a banana or other fruits.

• Breads and pastas made with whole-grain flour are important fiber sources. Multi-grain breads and whole-wheat pasta are fiber foods that are rich in flavor. Use brown rice instead of white rice. Make sandwiches with whole-wheat, bran, rye or other hearty, whole-grain breads. Pumpernickel and raisin bread are high in fiber. Make French toast from whole-grain breads. Make waffles or pancakes with whole-grain flours and top with fresh fruits and berries.

• Keep a supply of high-fiber convenience foods at work, at home, in suitcases, even in your car, so that fiber is always available.

Interestingly, foods that are consumed the same way they are grown, without additives or processing, such as most of the high-fiber sources, are naturally low in calories. For fiber content of specific foods, refer to Appendix A.

In summary, there are many theories as to why fiber helps in the prevention of colorectal cancer, including:

• Fiber increases stool bulk and therefore decreases the concentration of potentially harmful substances in the large bowel.

• Fiber seems to keep the stool soft, thus decreasing irritation to the large bowel during the solidifying, storing and excreting processes.

• Fiber may increase the speed at which waste materials move through the large bowel, giving cancer-causing agents less time to come into contact with colorectal cells.

• Fiber binds potentially harmful chemicals to itself and may neutralize possible negative effects on colorectal cells.

• Some types of fiber may increase the activity of bacteria in the large bowel. This leads to the production of substances that may protect the large bowel against cancerous changes.

17

Fruits & Vegetables

For flavor, color and texture, no group of foods lends greater variety to an eating program than fruits and vegetables. That's just the beginning. Fruits and vegetables are also rich in vitamins and minerals, low in fat and comparatively high in dietary fiber. Many scientists believe two categories of vegetables and fruits contain substances that help protect against the development of cancer.

One category is comprised of *green leafy vegetables; red, yellow and orange vegetables and fruits; citrus fruits;* and *fruit and vegetable juices.* These are good sources of vitamin A, vitamin C and beta carotene, a substance that the body converts to vitamin A.

The most beneficial members of the first category are Swiss chard, kale, spinach, romaine, endive, chicory, escarole, watercress, asparagus, green and red peppers, bean sprouts, mushrooms, squash, green beans, onions, okra, tomatoes and collard.

Also good are yellow-orange vegetables such as carrots, sweet potatoes, pumpkins and winter squash; and yellow-orange fruits such as apricots, cantaloupes, cherries, papayas and peaches. Although they are not yellow in all forms, berries, pineapples, plums, prunes, strawberries and watermelons are included in the yellow-orange category. Citrus fruits include lemons, limes, oranges, tangerines and grapefruits. Juices made from all these fruits and vegetables complete this category.

The second category of potential cancer-reducing foods is vegetables in the *mustard family*. These *cruciferous* vegetables are a good source of fiber and vitamins and include bok choy, broccoli, Brussels sprouts, cabbage, cauliflower, collard, kale, kohlrabi, mustard greens, turnips, turnip greens and rutabagas.

There appears to be more evidence for a cancer-protective effect from vegetables than from fruits.

The National Cancer Institute recommends eating a variety of these vitamin-rich foods rather than relying on vitamin and mineral supplements. It is recommended that everyone eat a minimum of four servings of fruits and vegetables daily. Sample one-serving sizes include 1/2 cup of cut vegetables or fruits, 1/2 medium-size grapefruit or melon, one bowl of salad, one orange or one medium potato. Single-serving sizes are further defined in the lists in Appendix A.

Fresh and frozen fruits and vegetables have more nutrients than the same foods canned. When fresh products cannot be obtained, the first alternative should be frozen ones. These require only a blanching—dipping in boiling water for one or two minutes before packaging. This helps to maintain their texture, flavor and nutritional value—qualities that are diminished when foods are canned. If you must buy canned goods, look for vegetables without added salt and fruits packed in juice rather than syrup. Avoid eating fruits and vegetables packaged in rich sauces. They are high in fat, salt and calories.

Fresh vegetables and fruits that have been picked unripe and stored for weeks or that have been kept unrefrigerated lose part of their nutritional value. Likewise, long storage in the home refrigerator leads to loss of nutrients. The best advice is to shop often for fresh fruits and vegetables, buying just enough to last a few days. When storage or timeliness of purchase becomes a concern, it may be better to buy frozen versions of the same products. These are typically picked when ripe and processed soon thereafter, preserving valuable nutrients.

The most nutritious way to eat fruits and vegetables is raw. Do not "soak" fresh fruits or vegetables. Rinse, drain, dry and then refrigerate fresh fruits and vegetables. Do not cut them up until they are going to be consumed. If they must be prepared in advance, seal them in plastic bags and refrigerate.

Avoid boiling vegetables in water. Microwave, bake, pressure cook or steam them instead. Boiling flushes nutrients into the water, which is usually thrown away. However, boiling vegetables in soups and stews is an excellent way to retain the nutrients.

Eating fruits and vegetables is recommended by the National Institutes of Health, the American Cancer Society and a multitude of other organizations dedicated to cancer prevention. Many other agencies endorse their consumption as well. The U.S. Department of Agriculture, American Heart

Association, National Academy of Sciences, U.S. Surgeon General and American Diabetic Association recommend fresh, canned, frozen, cooked or dried fruits and vegetables for reducing the risk of heart disease, strokes, diabetes and obesity.

Fruits and vegetables are recognized as important sources for vitamins A, C and E. These vitamins fall into a classification of chemical compounds known as *antioxidants*. Although oxygen is essential for sustaining life, the body's oxidation process produces chemical compounds called *free radicals* that have been linked to the development of cancer. Human cells have a built-in system that naturally fights free radicals but the body theoretically needs additional antioxidant power to neutralize the free radicals. Beta carotene, vitamin C and especially vitamin E are believed to have potent antioxidant capabilities that will block free radicals from doing damage.

The following guide to fruits and vegetables was distributed by the PPT. This material is adapted from information supplied by the United Fresh Fruit and Vegetable Association.

For further information on fruits and vegetables, refer to Appendix A.

Guide to Fruits and Vegetables

Fruits

Apples—Select fruits that have good color and feel firm to the touch. Skins should be smooth and free from bruises. If buying apples pre-packed in plastic bags, inspect them to ensure good quality. Handle apples carefully to prevent bruising. Store in a plastic bag in the refrigerator. Warm temperatures cause apples to lose crispness and flavor.

Apricots—Look for deep-yellow or yellowish-orange fruits that are plump and fairly firm. Avoid those that are soft, very firm, yellow or greenish-yellow. Allow apricots to ripen at room temperature until they yield to gentle palm pressure. Store fully ripened fruits in the refrigerator.

Bananas—Bananas arrive at the market at different stages of ripeness, so make your selection based on how and when you plan to use them. Ripen at room temperature to the desired stage, then use or refrigerate. Fully ripe bananas will keep in the refrigerator for a few days. The skin will darken but the fruit inside is fine.

Blueberries—Look for plump, fresh berries with a delicate, powdery coating. They should be purple to pale blue in color. Avoid baskets of berries that leak juice. Keep them covered and refrigerated. If in good condition, blueberries will keep in the refrigerator one week or more. Do not rinse until ready to use.

Cantaloupes—Choose well-shaped fruits completely covered with a netting over a creamy white or yellow background. Look for a smooth, rounded area at the stem end. A fragrant aroma is a good sign of a ripe fruit. A ready-to-eat melon gives slightly when pressed at the stem end. Store unripe melons at room temperature.

Casaba Melons—The skin of a casaba is golden yellow when ripe. Keep at room temperature until ripe, then refrigerate.

Cherries—Sweet cherries should be plump, firm and brightly colored. Colors range from red, yellow tinged with red and reddish-brown to black, depending on variety. Cherries are ready-to-eat when you buy them. Keep them refrigerated and use within a few days.

Cranberries—Select plump, firm, lustrous red to reddish-black berries. Refrigerate and use within two weeks. Can be stored in freezer in the original package for up to one year.

Crenshaw Melons—When ripe, a crenshaw melon has a golden rind that is sometimes tinged with green. Skin can be smooth or slightly ribbed. Keep at room temperature until the melon gives slightly at the stem end when gently pressed.

Grapefruit—For the juiciest grapefruit, look for a firm, well-shaped fruit that is heavy for its size. Skin that is blemished or tinged green does not affect the fruit's flavor or quality.

Grapes—Grapes are shipped from growers ready-to-eat, so enjoy them immediately for best flavor. Select well-formed bunches with fruit that is plump and has good color. Avoid bunches containing dry and brittle stems or sticky fruit. Store grapes in refrigerator in plastic bags. Rinse grapes under a gentle spray of water just before serving.

Honeydew Melons—Select those with smooth, velvety rinds that are creamy-white or yellow. Avoid fruits with stark white rinds tinged with green. Melon is ripe when rind gives slightly when gently pressed at blossom end. A fragrant aroma is another sign of ripeness. If not ripe, keep at room temperature a few days, then refrigerate.

Kiwifruit—Select plump fruits. Keep hard, unripe fruits at room temperature a few days, until they yield to gentle palm pressure. Store in refrigerator when ripe.

Lemons and Limes—Look for fine-textured skin. The juiciest ones will be heavy for their size. Lemons and limes keep best if refrigerated but can be stored at room temperature.

Mangos—Fruits vary in size, shape and color, depending on the variety. They may be oval, round or kidney-shaped. When ripe, skin color can be yellow, green or red, depending on the variety. To decide whether green ones are ripe, check that they are soft. Store mangos at room temperature until ripe, then refrigerate.

Nectarines—Choose plump, well-formed fruits. Some varieties are slightly blushed with crimson; others are almost all red. Look for cream to yellow background color without any green. For best flavor, eat when fully ripe. Once ripe, nectarines should be refrigerated and used promptly.

Oranges—Select firm fruits that are heavy for their size, which indicates juiciness. Sometimes skins are blemished or tinged with green but this does not affect fruit quality. For optimum storage life, keep oranges refrigerated.

Papayas—Green skin turns golden yellow as it ripens. Keep at room temperature until skin becomes mostly yellow. Ripe fruit gives to gentle pressure at the large end. Refrigerate when ripe. Flesh color can be yellow or orange when ripe.

Peaches—Select plump, well-shaped peaches with a creamy or golden undercolor. The red blush indicates variety and is not a sign of ripeness. Avoid fruits tinged with green because they often do not ripen completely. Ripen fruits at room temperature until they yield to gentle palm pressure.

Persian Melons—Dark-green undercolor turns a lighter green as the melon ripens. When ready-to-eat, the melon will give slightly to gentle pressure at the stem end. Store at room temperature for a few days if not ripe.

Pineapples—Select large fruits that have fresh green leaves. Shell can be either green or golden, which indicates variety, not ripeness. The best sign of freshness is a distinctive aroma. For best flavor, refrigerate before eating. Pineapples don't ripen further after they are picked, so use them as soon as possible.

Plums—Choose from a rainbow of colors with tastes ranging from tart to sweet, depending on the variety. Store plums at room temperature until ripe, then refrigerate and eat as soon as possible.

Pomegranates—Look for large fruits that feel heavy for their size. Generally, rinds are a deep, rich red but color can vary. Refrigerated, fruits will keep for several weeks.

Strawberries—Choose fruits that are bright red with fresh green caps. Keep refrigerated with caps attached until ready to use. Use as soon as possible for best quality. Rinse berries gently under cool running water just before eating.

Tangelos and Tangerines—Choose fruit heavy for its size. A puffy appearance is normal. For best flavor keep refrigerated.

Watermelons—Choose firm smooth melons with rinds that have a waxy bloom or dullness. Underside should be yellowish or creamy white. Avoid fruits with stark white or greenish undersides. When selecting cut melons, look for red, juicy flesh with black or dark brown seeds. Avoid melons with white streaks, white seeds and pale-colored flesh. Store uncut melons at room temperature or refrigerate. Cover and refrigerate cut melons.

Vegetables

Artichokes—Choose compact, heavy, plump, olive-green globes with large, tightly clinging leaf scales. Bronze tinge does not affect quality. Size is not an important quality factor.

Asparagus—Spears should be fresh and trim with closed compact tips. Select spears that have a large amount of green color.

Beans, Snap—Pods should be firm, crisp and slender, with good green color.

Broccoli—Look for compact bud clusters. Color varies from dark green to purplish green, depending on variety. Yellowing, wilted leaves and loose clusters indicate buds are past their prime.

Brussels Sprouts—Select those that are firm and compact with bright leaves. Avoid wilted or yellow leaves.

Cabbage—Heads should be reasonably solid and heavy in relation to size. Color, whether green or red, should not be dull.

Carrots—Select firm, well-shaped, bright orange roots.

Cauliflower—White or creamy-white, firm, compact curds indicate quality. Size of head bears no relation to quality.

Celery—Choose fresh crisp stalks that are thick and solid with good heart formation.

Corn, Sweet—Select only corn that is cold to the touch. Husks should be green, not dry or yellowish.

Cucumbers—Look for medium-size fruits with rich green color. Avoid large, puffy vegetables or those tinged with yellow.

Eggplant—Choose those that are firm and heavy for their size, with dark purple to purple-black skin.

Endive, Escarole and Chicory—Heads should be fresh, clean, crisp and cool to the touch. Avoid heads with dry, yellowish or wilted leaves, or those showing reddish discoloration of the hearts.

Greens (Collards, Turnip, Beet, Kale)—Choose fresh, crisp green leaves. Avoid any with coarse stems or wilted, yellowing leaves.

Kohlrabi—Stems should be medium-size, firm and crisp with crisp green tops.

Leeks—Select well-blanched bunches. White coloring should extend two to three inches from bulb base. Small to medium leeks are the most tender. Refrigerate in a plastic bag and use within three to five days.

Lettuce, Iceberg—Heads should be firm but give slightly when squeezed. At home, core the head by whacking it core-end down on the kitchen counter. Twist to remove the core and rinse under cold running water. Place core-end down in colander or rack and allow to drain thoroughly. Store in a tightly closed plastic bag or lettuce crisper.

Lettuce (Romaine, Boston, Bibb, Leaf)—Select clean, fresh and tender heads. Store in a tightly closed plastic bag or lettuce crisper.

Mushrooms—White, tan and cream-colored varieties are available. Freshest mushrooms are closed around the stem by a thin veil. Those having open veils (caused by loss of water) are just as nutritious but have a more pungent flavor. Refrigerate in a paper bag or ventilated plastic container. Do not store in closed plastic bags.

Okra—Pods should be young and tender, preferably two inches to four inches long. Avoid dull, dry or shriveled pods.

Onions—Choose onions that are clean and firm. Skins should be dry, smooth and crackly. Signs of decay include wet, soggy necks and soft or spongy bulbs. Keep in cool, well-ventilated area. May be refrigerated, but must be kept dry. They can be stored three to four weeks.

Onions, Green—Select young and tender bunches with fresh green tops. Keep refrigerated in a plastic bag. Use as soon as possible.

Parsnips—Select smooth, firm, well-shaped parsnips of small to medium size. Discoloration may be an indication of freezing.

Peppers—Select fresh, firm and thick-fleshed peppers, with bright coloring. They may be green, yellow or red. Immature peppers are usually soft with a dull color.

Potatoes—Choose firm, clean and relatively smooth potatoes free of cuts or bruises. Avoid those with green coloration and those with sprouts. Never refrigerate potatoes. Store in a cool, dark, well-ventilated area. Keep away from moisture and light, which can cause greening.

Radishes—A variety of sizes and shapes are available. All should be fresh, smooth and well-formed, without cuts, pits or black spots. Avoid spongy radishes.

Rhubarb—Select bright, crisp and firm stalks of medium size. Oversized stalks may be tough. Darker red stalks are generally more flavorful, but this does not always indicate quality. Store refrigerated in plastic bag.

Rutabagas—Should be firm, smooth and heavy for size. Avoid those with deep cuts or punctures. Size is not a quality factor.

Spinach—Leaves should be clean, fresh and dark green. Avoid bunches with large yellow leaves or leaves that are wilted or discolored.

Squash, Soft-skinned (Summer Squash: includes yellow crook-neck and zucchini)—Choose small to medium squash that feel heavy for their size. Refrigerate and use as soon as possible.

Squash, Hard-shelled (Winter Squash)—Avoid vegetables with soft spots. Hubbard squash can be stored six months or longer. Acorn squash can be stored three to six months. Don't refrigerate. Store in dry, well-ventilated area at room temperature.

Sweet Potatoes—Look for sweet potatoes with evenly colored and blemish-free skins. Select those that are firm and well-shaped, tapering at both ends. Handle gently to avoid bruising. Do not refrigerate. Store in cool, dry, well-ventilated area.

Tomatoes—Choose smooth, firm, plump tomatoes with bright color. Those purchased at the market usually require further ripening at home. Store at room temperature, away from direct sunlight. Place in a paper bag to hasten ripening. Best flavor if never refrigerated.

Turnips—Select firm smooth turnips of medium size. Avoid those with yellowed or wilted tops, which indicate aging.

18

Conclusions

This book's medical information consists of the explanations I went searching for soon after being advised I had cancer. I was dissatisfied with my doctor's brief and incomplete reasons for performing strange procedures in my body. I am not comfortable with any situation that is out of my control. I wanted to gain an understanding so I could make intelligent decisions. This illness was affecting my body—not the doctor's—and I didn't like being in the dark.

I am not sure of the value or benefits that can be derived from the personal narrative in the prologue to this book. Yet, as I reviewed all the research material in the context of my diary, I was struck with one undeniable fact: *My reactions to cancer were not unique*. In retrospect, I regret most not sharing my burden with loved ones from the very beginning, as my emotional roller-coaster traveled from thoughts of death to dedicating myself to fighting back my illness. Many new cancer patients try to deny or hide the diagnosis and to grapple alone with the emotional ramifications of the disease. On-again/off-again depression mixed with attempts to overcome feelings of self-pity are normal types of behavior for people confronting a mysterious, frightening cancer.

The Prologue and Section I of this book are the result of my natural reactions to a totally unexpected turn of events in my life. But the diet-related material created by PPT supplied the ultimate motivation to bring everything together in book form. The PPT provided me and 1000 or so other participants from around the United States with an opportunity to take responsive actions.

But what about the million other people who are advised every year that they have polyps? And what course should the 150,000 people who are annually diagnosed with colorectal cancer take? The material in this book supplies no secret cures or formulas. But it does provide the tools to fight back. Good luck in your quest!

Appendix A

High-Fiber, Lowfat Food Lists

Table of Contents

A Few Words About Implied Endorsement

The following lists were adapted from materials prepared for use in the Polyp Prevention Trials. Use of brand names in no way implies endorsement of the products by the National Cancer Society, the author or the publisher. Nutritional information is up-to-date at the time of printing, but may change at any time. Read the label information on the product for the currently correct figures. The product names shown are trademarked or registered, but we have not shown ® or ™ with the product names.

High-Fiber, Lowfat Foods

	Serving Size	Fiber Grams	Fat Grams
Breads			
Arnolds Bran'nola Original	1 slice	3	1
Arnolds Bran'nola Dark Wheat	1 slice	3	1
Diet Bread w/Fiber Added	2 slices	5	1
(Less or Taystee Lite)			
Earth Grains Lite 35 White	1 slice	4	1
Iverson Russian Rye	1 slice	3	1
Pita Bread, Whole Wheat,	1	6	1
6-1/2" diam.			
Roman Meal Light	1 slice	3	1
Oat Bran & Honey			
Stroehmann Whole White Bread	1 slice	4	1
Whole Wheat Bread, Mixed Grain,			
Wheat Germ, Granola Type	1 slice	2	1
Wonder Wheat Light	1 slice	2	0
Wonder High Fiber Wheat	1 slice	3	0
Muffins, Bagels and Waffles			
Arrowhead Mills Muffin Mixes			
Oat Bran Apple Spice	1	4	4
Wheat Bran	1	4	4
Aunt Jemima Pancake & Waffle Mix			
Buckwheat, 4" pancakes	3	5	2
Whole-Wheat, 4" pancakes	3	4	1
Aunt Jemima frozen			
whole-grain waffles	2	3	3
Belgian Chef Oat-Bran Waffle	1	6	3
Health Valley Fat-Free Muffins			
Almond Date Oat Bran	1	8	0
Apple Spice	1	5	0
Banana	1	5	0
Blueberry-Apple Oat Bran	1	5	0
Blueberry Oat Bran	1	8	0
Carrot Multi-Bran	1	5	0

	Serving Size	Fiber Grams	Fat Grams
Raisin Oat Bran	1	8	0
Raisin Spice	1	5	0
Raspberry Multi-Bran	1	5	0
Pepperidge Farms Healthy Choice			
Cinnamon Raisin Bran			
English Muffin	1	4	1
Country White English Muffin	1	2	1
Apple Oatmeal Muffin	1	3	4
Blueberry Muffin	1	2	2
Raisin Bran Muffin	1	4	2
Van's Belgian Waffles			
Oat Bran & Raisin	1	4	4
7-Grain	1	4	2
Van's Toaster Waffles			
Apple Cinnamon	1	3	3
Honey Almond	1	3	3
Multi-Grain	1	3	3
Sara Lee Deli-Style Oat-Bran Bagels	1	3	1
Washington Muffin Mixes			
(egg-white directions)			
Bran	1	2	3
Oat Bran and Cinnamon	1	4	4
Multi-Bran	1	5	3
Wonder High Fiber English Muffin	1	5	1

Crackers

	Serving Size	Fiber Grams	Fat Grams
Ralston Ry-Krisp Naturals	2	4	0
Ralston Ry-Krisp Sesame	2	3	1
Ryvita High Crispbread	2	4	0
Ryvita Sesame Rye Crispbread	2	3	1
Wasa Fiber Plus	1	3	1
Wasa Hearty Rye Crispbread	1	2½	0
Wasa Lite Rye Crispbread	2	2½	0
Wasa Sesame Crispbread	1	3	1

	Serving Size	Fiber Grams	Fat Grams
Breakfast Bars/Granola Bars			
Natural Nectar FI-BARs			
Apple-Oatmeal Spice	1	5	3
Raisin Nut Bran	1	5	4
Strawberry-Oatmeal & Almond	1	5	4
Cranberry & Wild Berries, Raspberry, & Strawberry	1	4	2
Granola Bar-Peanut Butter,Coconut	1	6	4
Slim Fast Bar			
Dutch Chocolate	1	6	4
Vanilla Almond Crunch	1	3	4
Cereals			
100% Bran	½ cup	10	1
Amaranth Cereal	½ cup	5	4
Benefit Cereal	1 cup	6	2
Bran Flakes	1 cup	6	0
Bran Muffin Crisp	1 cup	6	1
Corn Bran	1 cup	5	1
Crunchy Bran	1 cup	5	1
Fiber 7 Flakes	1 cup	5	1
Lightly Frosted Bran	¾ cup	3	0
Oat Squares	1 cup	5	2
Oat Bran Ready-to-Eat Cereal	¾ cup	4	2
Raisin Bran Cereal	¾ cup	5	1
General Mills Fiber One	½ cup	13	1
General Mills Total or Wheaties	¾ cup	3	1
General Mills Total Raisin Bran	1 cup	5	1
Health Valley 10 Bran Cereal	1 oz.	5	<1
Health Valley Natural Bran			
With Raisins	1 cup	18	3
With Apples & Cinnamon	1 cup	18	3
Health Valley Oat Bran Flakes	1 cup	5	2

	Serving Size	Fiber Grams	Fat Grams
Kellogg's 40% Bran Flakes	¾ cup	5	0
Kellogg's All-Bran	½ cup	9	1
Kellogg's All-Bran			
With Extra Fiber	½ cup	14	1
With Fruit & Almonds	½ cup	8	2
Kellogg's Bran Buds	½ cup	8	1
Kellogg's Common Sense			
Oat Bran	1 cup	5	1
Kellogg's Common Sense Oat Bran			
with Raisins	1 cup	7	2
Kellogg's Frosted Mini-Wheats	4 pieces	3	0
Kellogg's Fruitful Bran	¾ cup	5	0
Fruit Wheats, All Flavors	1 cup	6	0
Kellogg's Heartwise	1 cup	8	1
Kellogg's Nutri-Grain Wheat	¾ cup	3	0
Kellogg's Raisin Bran	¾ cup	5	1
Mueslix Bran Cereal	1 cup	7	4
Mueslix Five-Grain Cereal	1 cup	7	4
Nabisco Shredded			
Wheat 'N' Bran	¾ cup	4	1
Nabisco Wholesome 'N' Hearty	¾ cup	5	1
Nutri-Grain Nuggets	½ cup	8	1
Nutri-Grain Wheat & Raisin Bran	1 cup	5	1
Post Grape Nuts	½ cup	5	0
Post Shredded Wheat	1 cup	5	5
Pritikin Hearty Hot Cereal	1 packet	5	1
Quaker Crunchy Bran Cereal	¾ cup	6	1
Ralston Oat Bran	1 cup	3	1
Ralston Multibran Chex	1¼ cup	7	1
Ralston Wheat Chex	¾ cup	4	0
Roman Meal Cereal	1 cup	10	1
Uncle Sam's High Fiber	1 cup	5	4
Wheatena	½ cup	4	1

	Serving Size	Fiber Grams	Fat Grams
Flours, Grain and Pasta			
Barley, cooked	1 cup	9	1
Bulgur, cooked	1 cup	12	1
Oat bran, dry	1 cup	14	7
Oatmeal, dry	1 cup	8	5
Rye flour, medium	1 cup	15	2
Whole wheat flour	1 cup	13	2
Whole wheat macaroni, cooked	1 cup	5	1
Fruits			
Apples, dehydrated	¼ cup	2	<1
Apples, raw with skin	1 medium	3	<1
Applesauce, canned	½ cup	2	<1
Bananas, raw	1 medium	2	<1
Blackberries, canned, in syrup	½ cup	3½	<1
Blackberries, raw	½ cup	3½	<1
Blueberries, canned in syrup	½ cup	2½	<1
Blueberries, raw	½ cup	2½	<1
Boysenberries, canned, syrup or water pack	½ cup	3½	<1
Boysenberries, frozen, unsweetened	½ cup	3½	<1
Cantaloupe, fresh, 6" diameter	½	3½	<1
Cherries, sour, canned	½ cup	1½	<1
Dates, dried	½ cup	5	<1
Elderberries, raw	½ cup	3½	<1
Figs, dried	½ cup	9	1
Figs, canned, heavy syrup	1 cup	8	<1
Fruit cocktail, canned in syrup	½ cup	2	<1
Fruit cocktail, canned in water	½ cup	1½	<1
Gooseberries, raw	½ cup	3	<1
Grapefruit sections, canned, juice pack	½ cup	½	<1

	Serving Size	Fiber Grams	Fat Grams
Grapefruits, raw	½ medium	2	<1
Grapes, raw	½ cup	½	<1
Honeydew melon, 7" diameter	½	6	<1
Kiwi fruit	2 medium	5	<1
Mango	1 medium	2	1
Nectarines, raw	1 medium	2	1
Oranges, mandarin, canned, juice pack	½ cup	1½	0
Oranges, raw	1 medium	3	<1
Papayas, raw	½ cup	2	0
Peaches, canned, water pack, slices	½ cup	2	<1
Peaches, dried, uncooked	6 halves	6	1
Peaches, raw	1 medium	1½	<1
Pears, dried, uncooked	3 halves	6	1
Pears, raw	1 medium	4½	1
Pears, sweetened, cooked	½ cup	4	<1
Persimmons, Japanese, raw	1 medium	3	0
Pineapple, canned, chunks, juice pack	½ cup	2	<1
Pineapple, dried	½ cup	5	<1
Plums, canned, syrup pack	½ cup	3	<1
Plums, raw	1 medium	1	1
Pomegranate, fresh	1 medium	10	1
Prunes, dried, cooked	½ cup	7	<1
Raisins	¼ cup	2	<1
Raspberries, black or red, raw	½ cup	3	<1
Raspberries, frozen or canned, sweetened	½ cup	6	<1
Rhubarb, stewed, unsweetened	1 cup	6	0
Strawberries, raw	½ cup	2	<1
Tangerines, raw	1 medium	½	<1
Watermelon	½ cup	½	1

	Serving Size	Fiber Grams	Fat Grams
Legumes			
Baked beans with pork and tomato sauce	1 cup	14	3
Baked beans with pork and brown sugar	1 cup	14	4
Black beans, cooked, no fat added	1 cup	15	1
Blackeyed peas, fresh, cooked	1 cup	6	1
Blackeyed peas, canned	1 cup	16	1
Chickpeas, cooked or canned, no fat added	1 cup	10	4
Garbanzo beans, cooked, no fat added	1 cup	10	4
Health Valley Baked Beans	7.5 oz.	5	1
Kidney beans, cooked, no fat added	1 cup	11	1
Lentils, cooked, no fat added	1 cup	10	1
Lima beans, cooked, fresh or frozen	1 cup	9	1
Lima beans, cooked, no fat added	1 cup	14	1
Navy beans, cooked, no fat added	1 cup	15	1
Northern beans, cooked, no fat added	1 cup	10	1
Pinto beans, cooked, no fat added	1 cup	12	1
Refried beans, canned	1 cup	13	3
Soybeans, mature, cooked	½ cup	2	4
Split peas, cooked or canned, no fat added	1 cup	10	1

	Serving Size	Fiber Grams	Fat Grams
Soups			
Health Valley Soups and Chilis			
Black Bean	7.5 oz.	17	<1
Lentil	7.5 oz.	15	<1
Split Pea	7.5 oz.	13	<1
Mild BB Chili	5.0 oz.	12	<1
3-Bean Chili	5.0 oz.	9	<1
Pritikin Soups			
Tomato, with tomato pieces	1½ cup	6	0
Split Pea	1½ cup	8	0
Lentil	1½ cup	8	0
Navy Bean	1 cup	9	<1
Rokeach Soups			
Seven Bean	7.5 oz.	8	1
Vegetables			
Artichokes, including hearts, cooked	½ cup	3	<1
Asparagus, fresh or canned	½ cup	3	<1
Beans, green, cut, cooked	½ cup	2	<1
Beet greens, cooked, leaves and stems	½ cup	2	<1
Beets, cooked, sliced	½ cup	2	<1
Beets, pickled, canned, sliced	½ cup	2	<1
Broccoli, chopped, fresh or frozen, cooked	½ cup	2½	1
Brussels sprouts, fresh or frozen, cooked	½ cup	3½	1
Cabbage, green or red, cooked	½ cup	1½	<1
Carrot, raw	1 medium	2½	<1
Carrots, fresh or canned, cooked, sliced	½ cup	2½	<1
Cauliflower, fresh or frozen, cooked	½ cup	2½	<1

	Serving Size	Fiber Grams	Fat Grams
Collards, fresh or frozen, cooked	½ cup	2	<1
Corn, whole kernel, fresh or frozen	1 cup	6	<1
Corn, sweet, canned or frozen, cooked	½ cup	1½	1
Corn, sweet, canned, cream-style	½ cup	1½	4
Corn, ear	6" length	5	1
Cucumbers, raw, sliced	½ cup	½	<1
Dandelion greens, raw	1 cup	2	<1
Eggplant, cooked	½ cup	1	<1
Endive, raw, chopped	1 cup	1½	<1
Kale, fresh or frozen, cooked	½ cup	2	<1
Kohlrabi, raw	1 cup	5	<1
Leeks, raw, chopped	½ cup	1	<1
Lettuce, iceberg	1 cup	½	<1
Lettuce, romaine, chopped	1 cup	½	<1
Mixed vegetables (corn, lima beans, snap beans, peas and carrots)	½ cup	3	<1
Mushrooms, canned, drained	½ cup	1½	0
Mustard greens, chopped frozen, cooked	½ cup	2	<1
Okra, cooked, fresh or frozen	1 cup	6	1
Onions, fresh, cooked	½ cup	1½	
Parsnips, cooked, fresh or frozen	1 cup	6	1
Peas, fresh, canned or frozen, cooked	½ cup	3	<1
Peas and carrots	½ cup	3	<1
Potato, boiled, with skin	½ cup	2	<1
Potato, baked, with skin	1 medium	3	<1
Potato, baked, without skin	1 medium	2	<1

	Serving Size	Fiber Grams	Fat Grams
Potatoes, canned	1 cup	5	<1
Pumpkin, cooked, canned	1 cup	7	1
Sauerkraut, canned	½ cup	4	0
Scallion, cooked	1 cup	6	<1
Spinach, chopped, cooked	½ cup	2	
Squash, summer, cooked	½ cup	1½	<1
Squash, winter, all varieties, frozen, cooked	½ cup	3½	<1
Sweet potato, cooked, w/o skin	½ cup	4	<1
Sweet potatoes, candied or mashed	½ cup	1	0
Swiss chard, cooked	½ cup	2	<1
Tomato, raw	1 medium	1½	<1
Tomatoes, whole, canned	½ cup	1	<1
Tomato paste, canned	½ cup	6	1
Turnip greens, fresh or frozen, cooked	½ cup	2	<1
Turnips, fresh, cooked	½ cup	1½	0

Mixed Dishes

	Serving Size	Fiber Grams	Fat Grams
A La Crust			
Make Your Own Pizza	1/4 pizza	8	3
Amy's Kitchen			
Mexican Tamale Pie	8 oz.	7	1
Fantastic			
Cajun Red Beans & Rice	10 oz.	9	2
Caribbean Black Beans & Rice	10 oz.	8	2
Cha-Cha Chili	10 oz.	14	2
Curried Lentils & Rice	10 oz.	8	2
Leapin' Lentils Over Couscous	10 oz.	9	1
Pinto Beans & Rice Mexicana	10 oz.	10	2
White Beans & Rice Italiano	10 oz.	8	2

	Serving Size	Fiber Grams	Fat Grams
Health Valley Fat-Free Fast Menu			
Amaranth with			
Garden Vegetables	5 oz.	6	0
Hearty Lentil with			
Garden Vegetables	5 oz.	10	0
Western Black Bean			
with Garden Vegetables	5 oz.	10	0
Health Valley Tofu Fast Menu			
Home Baked Organic Beans			
with Tofu Wieners	7.5 oz.	16	3
Organic Black Beans			
with Tofu Wieners	7.5 oz.	14	3
Organic Lentils			
with Tofu Wieners	7.5 oz.	15	3

Making Lowfat Choices

CHOOSE MORE OFTEN

Lower-Fat Poultry, Fish and Meat

- Chicken, turkey, Rock Cornish hens (without skin)
- Fresh, frozen seafood water-packed canned fish
- Reduced-fat luncheon meats such as turkey bologna and hot dogs
- Beef, veal, lamb and pork cuts with little or no visible fat, all fat trimmed

Lowfat or Skim-Milk Dairy Products

- Lowfat or skim milk, and buttermilk
- Lowfat or diet margarine
- Lowfat yogurt
- Skimmed evaporated milk, nonfat dry milk
- Lowfat cheese (ricotta, pot, farmer, cottage, mozzarella, cheeses made from skim milk), Parmesan (small amounts)
- No-fat cheeses
- Sherbet, frozen nonfat or lowfat yogurt, ice milk

CHOOSE LESS OFTEN

Higher-Fat Poultry, Fish and Meat

- Duck and goose
- Poultry with skin
- Frozen fish sticks tuna packed in oil
- Regular luncheon meats, sausage
- Beef, veal, lamb and pork cuts with marbling, fat not trimmed

High-Fat Dairy Products

- Whole milk
- Butter
- Yogurt made from whole milk
- Sweet cream, sour cream, half-and-half, whipped cream, imitation toppings
- Soft cheeses such as cream cheese, cheese spreads, Camembert, Brie
- Hard cheeses such as Cheddar, Swiss, bleu, American, jack
- Ice cream
- Coffee creamers (including nondairy)
- Cream sauces, cream soups

CHOOSE MORE OFTEN	CHOOSE LESS OFTEN
Fats and Oils	**Fats and Oils**
• Fat-free and lowfat salad dressings • Lowfat or diet margarine	• Vegetable and salad oils, shortening, lard, meat fats, salt pork, bacon • Mayonnaise and salad dressings • Margarine, butter • Gravies, butter sauces
Whole-Grain Products	**Refined Bakery and Snack Products**
• Whole-wheat crackers and English muffins, bran muffins, bagels; brown, rye, oatmeal, pumpernickel, bran and corn breads • Bran cereals, shredded wheat, whole-grain or whole-wheat flaked cereals • Foods made with whole-grain flours, such as waffles, pancakes, pasta, taco shells • Foods made with other whole grains, including barley, buckwheat groats, bulgur wheat • Popcorn, unbuttered	• Refined-flour breads, quick breads, biscuits, buns, croissants • Donuts, pies, pastries, cakes, cookies, brownies • Potato chips and snack crackers • Canned puddings, icings and candies made with butter, cream or chocolate • Granola • Croissants

CHOOSE MORE OFTEN

Fruits and Vegetables

All are good choices, especially:
- Apples, pears, apricots, bananas, berries, cantaloupes, grapefruit, oranges, pineapples, papayas, prunes, raisins
- Carrots, broccoli, potatoes, corn, cauliflower, Brussels sprouts, cabbage, celery, green beans, summer squash, green peas, parsnips, kale, spinach, other greens, yams, sweet potatoes, turnips
- All dried peas and beans

Food Preparation

- Baking, broiling, boiling, stewing (skim off fat), poaching, stir-frying, simmering, steaming
- Use nonstick cookware, minimal or no fat added
- Season vegetables with herbs, spices or lemon juice

CHOOSE LESS OFTEN

Fruits and Vegetables

- Fried vegetables, vegetables with cream, cheese, or butter sauce
- Avocados, olives

Food Preparation

- Batter frying and deep-fat frying, sautéing
- Use of fatty gravies and sauces
- Adding cream or butter to vegetables

Lowfat Substitutes for High-Fat Ingredients

Instead of these high-fat ingredients . . . Try these lowfat substitutes

1 oz. bitter chocolate (15g fat)	1 to 1½ tsp. chocolate extract (0g fat) 2 T. cocoa powder (3.6g fat)
1 T. coconut (3g fat)	1/2 tsp. coconut extract (0g fat)
1 oz. (2 T.) cream cheese (9.8g fat)	1 oz. farmer's or cottage cheese (1.2g fat) 1 oz. lowfat cream cheese (2 to 6g fat) 1 oz. 1%-fat cottage cheese (0.3g fat) 1 oz. 4%-fat cottage cheese (1.2g fat)
1 cup evaporated milk (19.1g fat)	1 cup evaporated skim milk (0.5g fat)

Greasing pans with shortening
   (4 to 8g fat)
	Nonstick vegetable spray or waxed paper
	   (0 to 2g fat)

1 cup heavy cream (88.1g fat)	3/4 cup skim milk plus 1/4 cup nonfat dry milk powder (0.3g fat) 1 cup evaporated skim milk (0.5g fat) 1 cup 1% milk (2.6g fat)

1 T. mayonnaise (11g fat)	1 T. lowfat or nonfat mayonnaise
	   (0 to 5g fat)
	1/2 T. lowfat mayonnaise plus 1/2 T.
	   nonfat yogurt (2.5g fat)

1/4 cup nuts (16 to 19g fat)	1/4 cup nugget-type cereal or
	   other crunchy cereal (corn flakes,
	   crisped rice) (0 to 0.4g fat)

1 T. oil, butter, margarine
   (11 to 14g fat)
	1½ to 2 tsp. oil, butter,
	   margarine (6 to 7g fat)
	1 T. lowfat butter substitute (0 to 0.3g fat)
	1 T. reduced-fat margarine (3 to 6g fat)

Instead of these high-fat ingredients . . . Try these lowfat substitutes

1 oz. semisweet chocolate (9g fat)	1 to 1½ tsp. chocolate extract plus 1 T. sugar (0g fat)
	2 T. cocoa plus 1 T. sugar (3.6g fat)
1 T. sour cream (2.9g fat)	1 T. nonfat or lowfat yogurt* (0 to 0.2g fat)
	1 T. nonfat or lowfat sour cream (0 to 1g fat)
	1 T. lowfat buttermilk (1g fat)
1/4 cup whipped cream (9.2g fat)	1/4 cup powdered whipped-topping mix made with skim milk (2g fat)
	1/4 cup whipped evaporated skim milk (0.1g fat)
	1/4 cup "lite" nondairy topping (2g fat)
1 cup whole milk (8.2g fat)	1 cup skim milk (0.4g fat)
	1 cup 1% milk (2.6g fat)
	1 cup evaporated skim milk (0.5g fat)
	1 cup nonfat or lowfat yogurt (0 to 3g fat)
1 cup whole-milk ricotta cheese (31.9g fat)	1 cup "light" ricotta (8g fat)
	1 cup part-skim ricotta (19.5g fat)
	1 cup small-curd 1%-fat cottage cheese (2.3g fat)
	1 cup small-curd 2%-fat cottage cheese (4.4g fat)
	1 cup small-curd 4%-fat cottage cheese (9.5g fat)
1 whole egg (5g fat)	2 egg whites (0g fat)
	1/4 cup egg substitute (0 to 4g fat)

*When adding yogurt to hot dishes, add as a last step. Occasionally, yogurt will separate. To prevent separation, add 1 tablespoon cornstarch per cup of yogurt.

Getting To Know Fish

Fish	Fat Grams (per oz., cooked)	Texture & Flavor	Cooking Substitutions+	Suggested Cooking Methods
Anchovy (fresh)*	1.2	soft, salty	herring, sardines	grill, pan-fry
Bass Fresh-water	1.2	firm, mild	halibut, grouper orange roughy, mahi mahi, perch	bake, grill, broil, poach, pan-fry, stir-fry
Sea	0.4	medium firm, mild	grouper	poach, bake, grill, pan-fry, broil, stew, stir-fry
Bluefish	1.2	dark meat, firm but flaky, distinctive flavor	mackerel, white fish, trout	broil, grill, bake
Carp	2.1	bony, with strong flavor	----------	pan-fry, bake
Catfish	1.2	medium firm, sweet	trout	bake, broil, grill, poach, pan-fry
Cod	0.4	firm but flaky white flesh, sweet, mild	flounder, haddock	poach, broil, bake, grill, pan-fry, use in soups and stews
Flounder	0.4	mild, flaky	halibut, sole	pan-fry, broil, bake
Grouper	0.4	firm, mild	sea bass, snapper, halibut, pike	pan-fry, grill, poach, broil, bake, good in stews and chowder

*Canned anchovies are packed in oil and are higher in fat (3 grams of fat per ounce). Use sparingly in salads or as a topping for pizza.
+Substitutions may not have the same number of fat grams as the fish listed.

Fish	Fat Grams (per oz., cooked)	Texture & Flavor	Cooking Substitutions+	Suggested Cooking Methods
Haddock	0.4	sweet, mild, soft, flaky	cod, flounder	bake, poach, broil
Halibut	0.4	medium firm, mild, sweet	grouper, cod, snapper turbot	grill, broil, poach, bake
Herring	3.4	salty, oily, firm	sardines, anchovies	grill, bake
Mackerel	3.4	flesh varies from white to red; oily with strong flavor	bluefish, trout, whitefish	broil, grill
Mahi Mahi	0.4	firm, white flesh, mild	snapper, ono, salmon, cod, trout	grill, poach, bake, broil
Ocean Perch	0.4	flaky, delicate flavor	snapper, orange roughy, cod	steam, pan-fry, bake, broil
Ono (Wahoo)	3.4	firm, white flesh, sweet but distinct flavor	tuna, swordfish, shark	grill, broil, bake
Orange Roughy	2.1	medium dense, very mild	sole, cod, snapper, flounder	pan-fry, broil, grill, bake, poach
Pike	0.4	medium firm but flaky	cod, snapper	poach, bake, grill, pan-fry
Red Snapper	0.4	medium firm, mild, sweet	grouper, halibut orange roughy, sole, cod	broil, grill, bake, stew, stir-fry

+Substitutions may not have the same number of fat grams as the fish listed.

Fish	Fat Grams (per oz., cooked)	Texture & Flavor	Cooking Substitutions+	Suggested Cooking Methods
Salmon		firm and pink,	whitefish, trout	poach, grill, broil,
Chum	1.2	distinctive		bake, pan-fry
Atlantic	2.1	flavor		
King	3.4			
Sockeye	3.4			
Shad	0.8	soft, rich	salmon, trout	bake, broil, grill, pan-fry
Shark	1.2	firm, mild flavor	swordfish, ono, tuna	grill, stew, stir-fry, bake, broil
Smelt	1.2	sweet, tender	herring, sardine	pan-fry
Sole	0.4	sweet, flaky	flounder	poach, pan-fry, bake, steam
Swordfish	1.2	firm, mild	ono, shark, tuna	grill, bake, broil
Trout				
Lake	2.1	rich, mild, firm flakes	other trout, salmon, catfish	pan-fry, poach, bake, steam
Rainbow	1.2	firm flakes, delicate flavor	salmon, other trout	pan-fry, poach, bake, steam
Tuna	1.2	firm, distinctive flavor	swordfish, shark, ono	grill, broil, poach, bake
Whitefish	1.2	white flesh, flaky, delicate, sweet, nutty	trout, salmon	bake, broil, grill, pan-fry

+Substitutions may not have the same number of fat grams as the fish listed.

Glorious Grains

Fat (g)	Fiber (g)	Description	Cooking Tips	Recipe Ideas
(per cooked cup)				
Amaranth				
3	8	Small cereal grain from a broad-leaf plant; slight peppery taste. Often sold in combination with other grains.	Use 1 cup grain to 3 cups water; simmer 1/2 to 3/4 hour or until tender. Can be popped like popcorn in a covered, ungreased skillet or wok. Seeds expand 3 to 4 times original size.	Use flour for breads, cakes and pancakes. Use seeds for pilaf, porridge or breakfast cereal.
Barley				
		Toasty, nutty flavor; chewy texture	Use 1 cup barley to 4 cups water.	Add to soups, casseroles or stews.
Whole 1	10	Whole: entire grain	Simmer 1¼ hours.	Use by itself with seasonings.
Pearl 1	5	Pearl: germ and bran layers removed	Simmer 45 minutes.	Mix with leftovers
Buckwheat Groats				
1	3	Rich brown color, nutty flavor, soft texture. Kasha is the roasted version and has a stronger flavor.	Use 1 cup buckwheat to 2 cups water. Simmer 15 to 30 minutes. Make flour by grinding uncooked grain in a food processor or blender until fine.	Makes good pilaf by itself or mixed with equal parts of bulgur or rice. Use in Russian dishes. Try flour in pancakes.
(Kasha)				
Bulgur				
1	12	Cracked wheat that has been hulled, steamed and dried. Nutty flavor with chewy texture. Available in 3 sizes (largest for pilaf, middle for cereal, smallest for tabouli). Also in tabouli mix.	Use 1 cup bulgur to 2 cups water. Simmer 15 to 20 minutes. Smaller (salad) size can be cooked by soaking in 1 to 2 cups boiling water per 1 cup bulgur for 10 to 15 minutes. Drain excess water before serving.	Serve like rice. Use in salads and side dishes. Use as a cereal.

Fat (g) Fiber (g) Description (per cooked cup)			Cooking Tips	Recipe Ideas

Cornmeal (polenta)

	1	2	Coarse or finely ground corn kernels (white or yellow). Sweet flavor with soft texture.	Use l cup cornmeal to 4 cups water. Simmer l /2 hour.	Use in polenta or as a cereal Finely ground meal can be used in muffins and breads.

Hominy

	1	4	Skinned white corn kernels; slightly sweet flavor; firm texture.	Use 1 cup hominy to 4 cups water; soak overnight; simmer 2 to 3 hours. Also available canned (precooked).	Use in side or main dishes or as a cereal.

Hominy grits

	1	1	Ground hominy; available in various textures from fine to coarse	Cook 1 cup grits with 4 cups water for 30 minutes. Quick cooking/instant varieties are also available.	Use in cereals and for baking breads, muffins, pancakes. Also good as a side dish or served with lowfat or nonfat cheese.

Couscous

	0	2	Flour-coated, finely cracked wheat that has been steamed and dried; bland, slightly nutty flavor	Use 1 cup couscous to 2 cups water; cook for 5 to 15 minutes (depending on the variety).	Serve like rice (in main and side dishes, in puddings, in salads); use as cereal.

Millet

	1	3	Small, round kernels; tan-colored; delicate, sweet, nutty flavor; chewy texture	Use 1 cup millet to 2½ cups water simmer for 30 to 45 minutes. Prepare just before eating as it solidifies as it cools; add leftovers to soup.	Serve millet like rice. Use in soups or add to chili. Good as an accompaniment to spicy dishes. Eat as a light breakfast cereal.

Oats

Oat Groats

	2	4	Whole kernel; nutty flavor; chewy texture; doesn't get mushy like oatmeal	Use 1 cup groats to 2 cups water; simmer for 1 hour. (Use 3 cups water for cereal.)	Serve as side dish or cereal.

Fat (g) Fiber (g) Description (per cooked cup)			Cooking Tips	Recipe Ideas

Oats (continued)

Oatmeal (rolled; quick-cooking; instant)

| 2 | 4 | Oat groats that have been steamed, then flattened, cut or flaked; old-fashioned and instant vary in coarseness of cut | Use 1 cup oatmeal to 1 to 1½ cups water (the greater the amount of water the creamier the results). Follow directions on package for cooking time. | Use as a cereal or in baked products such as cakes, cookies, muffins, and breads. |

Steel-cut Oats (Scottish or Irish)

| 2 | 4 | Sliced oat groats; nutty flavor and firm texture | Use 1 cup oats to 2 cups water; simmer for 30 minutes. | Use for cereals and for baking. |

Oat Bran

| 3 | 5 | Outer coating of the oat kernel; small brown flakes | Use 1 cup oat bran to 1 to 1½ cups water. Follow directions on package for cooking time. | Use as a cereal or in baked goods. Add to meatloaf, cereals, casseroles. |

Quinoa

| 3 | 2 | Small, round, pale-yellow seed; sweet and nutty in flavor; light, fluffy and pleasantly crunchy | Rinse well before cooking; use 1 cup quinoa to 2 cups water; simmer for 15 minutes. | Serve like rice or as a base for salads. Add to soups and stews. Use as a cereal. |

Rice

Aromatic long-grain rice (Basmati, Texmati, Lundberg Royal, Wehani, Gourmet, O'Della)

| 1 | 1 | Long, slender white, tan and brown grains; fragrant, delicate taste; fluffy texture | Rinse; use 1 cup rice to 1½ cups water; simmer for 15 to 30 minutes. | Use for casseroles, side dishes, main dishes; as a base for salads. |

Brown rice (instant; short-, medium- or long-grain)

| 2 | 3 | Rice with the bran layer intact (therefore high in fiber); nutty flavor and soft texture; chewier than white rice | Use 1 cup brown rice to 2 cups water. Non-instant varieties take 30 to 45 minutes to cook. Follow package instructions for instant. | Use for side dishes, pilafs, casseroles, main dishes, pudding desserts, as a base for salads. |

Fat (g)	Fiber (g)	Description (per cooked cup)	Cooking Tips	Recipe Ideas
Rice (continued)				
Italian short-grain rice (Arborio)				
1	1	Polished white kernels; rectangular shape; bland taste; soft texture	Use 1 cup rice to 2 cups water; simmer for 20 minutes.	Use in risotto recipes.
White rice (instant; short-, medium- or long-grain)				
1	1	Polished white kernels; bland flavor and firm texture	Use 1 cup rice to 2 cups water. Non-instant varieties take about 20 minutes to cook. Follow package directions for instant.	Use for casseroles, side dishes, pilafs, main dishes, pudding desserts, in soups, as a base for salads.
Wild rice				
1	2	Brown-colored; intense, nutty flavor; firm, chewy texture	Use 1 cup wild rice to 3 cups water; simmer for 45 minutes to 1 hour.	Use in salads, side dishes, pilafs, casseroles, mixed with white or brown rice, for stuffings.
Rye (whole rye berry or rye kernel)				
1	9	Sour flavor; soft texture	Use 1 cup rye kernels to 2 cups water; simmer for 45 minutes to 1 hour.	Use in cereals, stews, and breads. Use rye flour (light and dark) for breads, muffins, and pancakes.
Wheat				
Wheat Berries				
1	5	Unprocessed whole-wheat kernels; crunchy, nutty flavor; chewy texture (The ground whole-wheat kernel makes whole-wheat flour.)	Cook 1 cup wheat berries to 2 to 3 cups water for 1 to 1½ hours. No cooking needed when used in baking.	Use in salads and in baking. Use whole-wheat flour in baking

Fat (g) Fiber (g) Description (per cooked cup)			Cooking Tips	Recipe Ideas

Wheat (continued)

Wheat Bran+

3	26	Outer coating of the wheat seed; small brown flakes	No cooking needed.	Use in baking; as a topping; as a thickening agent. Add to meatloaf, cereals, muffins, pancakes. Use as a casserole topping.

Wheat, Cracked

1	5	Crushed whole-wheat kernels; hearty flavor; firm texture	Use 1 cup cracked wheat to 2 cups water; simmer for about 40 minutes. No cooking needed when used in baking.	Use in cereals and breads.

Wheat Germ+

12	16	Seed of the wheat kernel where much of the oil is found; small, brownish, round	No cooking needed. Can be purchased toasted.	Use in baking, as a topping, or as a thickening agent. Add to cereals. Sprinkle over yogurt, cottage cheese, fruits, vegetables. Use as a casserole topping.

+Fat and fiber values for wheat bran and wheat germ are for uncooked quantities

Bountiful Beans

Fat (g) Fiber (g) (per cooked cup)	Appearance & Taste	Availability	Cooking Tips (dry beans) Soak Simmer	Recipe Ideas
Chick peas (Garbanzo Beans or Ceci)				
4 10	Round, 3/8" diameter, beige. Nutty flavor with crunchy and soft texture.	dry or canned (precooked)	Yes 2 to 3 hours	Appetizers, salads, soups, casseroles, snacks by the handful. Purée for dips or soup thickeners.
Cranberry Beans (Roman Beans)				
1 12	Mottled cranberry red with ivory. Mealy texture with nutty flavor. Attractive pink color when cooked.	Dry	Yes 2 to 2½ hours	Succotash, salad, Italian and Portuguese dishes.
Fava Beans (Broad or Horse Beans)				
1 9	Flat oval, 3/4" diameter; creamy brown, with tough skin. Earthy flavor.	Dry or canned (precooked)	Yes l to l½ hours	Purées, salads and antipastos, mixed with other vegetables, in soups or stews, sautéed with garlic and herbs. Suited to Italian Greek or Spanish dishes.
Great Northern Beans (Haricot Beans)				
1 10	Kidney-shaped, 3/8" diameter; ivory-white. Delicate flavor and firm texture.	Dry or canned (precooked)	Yes 1½ to 2 hours	Boston baked beans, cassoulets, casseroles, soups, stews, main dishes, salads.
Kidney Beans				
1 11	Kidney-shaped, 1/2" long. Dark and light red Also available in black, brown and white varieties. Slightly sweet and meaty with mealy, soft texture.	Dry or canned (precooked)	Yes l to 2 hours	Salads (marinated or plain), casseroles, soups, chili, stews, Mexican dishes.

Fat (g)	Fiber (g)	Appearance & Taste	Availability	Cooking Tips (dry beans)		Recipe Ideas
(per cooked cup)				Soak	Simmer	
Lentils						
1	10	Small, flat, round, in green, brown, red or pink. Soft texture and mild earthy, nutty flavor.	Dry	No	/ to fl hour	Soups, salads (hot or cold), purées, stews, with rice or grains, in side or main dish casseroles, curry dishes.
Lima Beans (Butter Beans)						
1	14	Flat, oval, 1/2" (baby) to 1-1/4" (large) diameter. Light green. Soft and mealy with tough skin; mild taste, nutty flavor when eaten fresh; tender and sweet when cooked.	Fresh, dry, frozen or canned (precooked)	Yes	1 to 2 hours	Soups, side dishes, succotash, casseroles,stews purées.
Navy Beans						
1	15	Small, oval, white; interchangeable with Great Northern (Haricot) beans. Mealy texture and mild flavor.	Dry or canned (precooked)	Yes	1fi to 2fi hours	Soups, stews, purées, baked beans; take on the flavor of other foods and seasonings.
Pinto Beans						
1	12	Kidney-shaped, 3/8" long, beige with streaks of brownish pink. Mealy texture, mild earthy flavor.	Dry or canned (precooked)	Yes	2 to 2fi hours	Dips, Mexican dishes, stews, baked products.
Red Beans						
1	11	Medium, dark red, oval. Taste and texture similar to kidney beans.	Dry or canned (precooked)	Yes	2 to 3 hours	Soups, stews, with rice, Cajun dishes. Can be substituted for kidney beans.

Fat (g)	Fiber (g)	Appearance & Taste	Availability	Cooking Tips (dry beans) Soak	Simmer	Recipe Ideas
(per cooked cup)						
Soybeans						
15	4	Round, 3/8" diameter. Pale ivory, black, green or brown. Firm texture and bland flavor.	Dry or canned (precooked)	Yes	3 to 4 hours	Soups, stews. Often consumed processed as flour, bean curd (tofu) and soy sauce or tamari. These products are quite low in fat.
Split Peas						
1	10	Small halved peas, green or yellow. Mealy texture with earthy, nutty flavor	Dry or canned (precooked)	No	1/2 to 1 hr.	Appetizers, soups; with rice or grains.

Guide To Ethnic Foods

The following provides typical amounts of fat and fiber (rounded to whole numbers) in various ethnic restaurant dishes. Use these values only as a guide. Methods of preparation vary from restaurant to restaurant. If in doubt, ask how a dish is prepared before ordering.

	Serving Size	Fat (g)	Fiber (g)
Chinese			
Soups			
Egg Drop Soup	1 cup	4	0
Hot and Sour Soup	1 cup	7	1
Oriental Vegetable Soup	1 cup	3	1
Wonton Soup	1 cup	12	3
Fried Chow Mein Noodles	1 cup	14	2
Appetizers			
Chicken on a Stick	1 oz.	1	0
Egg Rolls, 4" long	1	11	1
Fried Wontons	1	4	0
Steamed Dumplings, Chicken or Seafood	1	3	0
Entrées			
Chop Suey, Chicken	1 cup	6	2
Chow Mein, Vegetable	1 cup	7	3
Egg Foo Yung, without meat, 4" diameter	1 piece	11	0
Lo Mein, Chicken	1 cup	7	1
Sweet and Sour Chicken	1 cup	21	2
Sweet and Sour Pork	1 cup	41	2
Yaka Mein	1 cup	8	2
Fried Rice	1 cup	14	2
Steamed Rice	1 cup	1	1
Vegetables			
Bamboo Shoots	1 cup	1	3
Bean Sprouts	1 cup	0	5
Snow Peas	1 cup	0	2
Water Chestnuts	1 cup	0	3
Sauces			
Black Bean Sauce	1 Tbsp	1	0
Hoisin Sauce	1 Tbsp	1	0
Lobster Sauce	1 Tbsp	2	0
Oyster Sauce	1 Tbsp	0	0

	Serving Size	Fat (g)	Fiber (g)
Plum Sauce	1 Tbsp	0	0
Sesame Oil	1 Tbsp	14	0
Sweet and Sour Sauce	1 Tbsp	0	0
Soy Sauce	1 Tbsp	0	0
Desserts			
Fortune Cookie	1	0	0
Lychee Nuts	1 cup	1	1
Mandarin Oranges, canned	1 cup	0	1
Pineapple Chunks, canned	1 cup	0	4

Italian

Appetizers and Side Dishes			
Antipasto Salad, no meat, cheese, or oil dressing	1 cup	0	1
Breadstick, Crisp	1 piece	2	0
Breadstick, Soft, 6-1/2" long	1	0	0
Italian Bread	1 slice	0	0
Minestrone Soup	1 cup	6	4
Pasta e Fagioli Soup	1 cup	7	3
Steamed Mussels in Tomato Sauce	3 oz.	3	0
Steamed Mussels in Wine Sauce	3 oz.	3	0
Entrées			
Eggplant Parmigiana	1 cup	25	3
Pasta, cooked			
white	1 cup	1	2
whole wheat	1 cup	1	5
vegetable	1 cup	2	3
Ravioli, Meat	1 cup	7	3
Shrimp Scampi	1 cup	22	1
Tortellini, Cheese	1 cup	14	2
Tortellini, Meat	1 cup	15	2
Veal Scallopine	1 cup	21	2
Meats			
Italian Sausage, 4" long	1	13	0
Mortadella	1 oz.	7	0
Pancetta, 0.2 oz. = 1 slice	1 slice	3	0
Pepperoni, 0.2 oz. = 1 slice	1 slice	2	0
Prosciutto	1 oz.	2	0
Sauces			
Alfredo Sauce	1/4 cup	12	0
Cacciatore Sauce	1/4 cup	7	1
Bolognese Sauce	1/4 cup	15	0

	Serving Size	Fat (g)	Fiber (g)
Marinara Sauce	1/4 cup	5	1
Marsala Sauce	1/4 cup	5	0
Red Clam Sauce	1/4 cup	2	1
White Clam Sauce	1/4 cup	3	0
Desserts			
Cappuccino	1 cup	3	0
Cappuccino with Skim Milk	1 cup	0	0
Italian Ice	1/2 cup	0	0

Mexican

	Serving Size	Fat (g)	Fiber (g)
Appetizers			
Tortilla Chips	1 cup	6	1
Salsa	1/4 cup	0	0
Guacamole	1/4 cup	5	2
Entrées			
Burrito, Bean, 3" long	1	5	4
Burrito, Beef, 3" long	1	25	2
Chicken Barbacoa	3 oz.	9	0
Chicken Fajita	1	9	2
Chimichanga, 5" long	1	18	5
Enchilada, Beef, Cheese, Bean, 5" long	1	14	3
Pechugo de Pollo,	3 oz. chicken, 1/2 cup vegetables	9	2
Quesadilla, Cheese (corn tortilla, baked)	1	20	2
Quesadilla, Cheese (corn tortilla, fried)	1	28	2
Quesadilla, Chicken (corn tortilla, baked)	1	5	2
Quesadilla, Chicken (corn tortilla, fried)	1	13	2
Taco, Bean, 4-3/4" long	1	13	4
Taco, Beef, 4-3/4" long	1	16	2
Tamale, 4" long	1	6	1
Tostada, with refried beans, 5-1/2" diameter	1	16	6
Side Dishes and Miscellaneous			
Refried Beans	1 cup	28	14
Vegetarian Refried Beans, lowfat	1 cup	3	13
Tortilla, Corn, plain, 5-1/2" diameter	1	1	1
Tortilla, Corn, fried, 5-1 /2" diameter	1	5	1
Tortilla, Flour, plain, 5-1/2" diameter	1	4	2
Tortilla, Flour, fried, 8" diameter	1	12	2

	Serving Size	Fat (g)	Fiber (g)
French			
Appetizers			
Consomme	1 cup	0	0
Salad (with no oil)	1 cup	0	1
Entrées/Sauces			
Bouillabaisse	1 cup	4	0
Bearnaise Sauce	¼ cup	27	0
Bechamel Sauce	¼ cup	8	0
Bordelaise Sauce	¼ cup	0	0
Hollandaise Sauce	¼ cup	27	0
Desserts			
Poached Pear	1 medium	1	4
Greek			
Appetizers and Dips			
Babaganoosh	1/4 cup	2	1
Greek Salad (with no oil)	1 cup	4	1
Hummus	1/4 cup	7	4
Pita Bread, Wheat, 6-1/2" diameter	1	1	6
Pita Bread, White, 6 -1/2" diameter	1	1	1
Tzateki	1 /4 cup	2	0
Entrées			
Gyro	1	10	1
Plaki	3 oz. fish with 1/4 cup sauce	8	1
Shish kabob with lamb	1 skewer	8	1
Desserts			
Baklava, 2" x 2"	1 piece	29	2
Extras and Miscellaneous			
Feta Cheese	1 oz.	6	0
Olives	2 medium	1	0
Phyllo (Filo) Dough, 3" x 2"	1 piece	0	0
Indian			
Appetizers, Breads, Soups			
Dal, Sambhar	1 cup	2	4
Nan, Pulka	1 piece	3	1

	Serving Size	Fat (g)	Fiber (g)
Entrées			
Biryani, Chicken	1 cup	10	2
Saag	1 cup	0	3
Seekh Kabob, Chicken or Fish	3 oz.	3	0
Tandoori Chicken	4 oz.	9	0
Extras and Miscellaneous			
Ghee	1 Tbsp	11	0
Paneer	2 oz.	3	0
Japanese			
Soups			
Miso Soup	1 cup	1	0
Entrées			
Beef Teriyaki	4 oz.	5	0
Shrimp Tempura	1 cup	22	1
Extras and Miscellaneous			
Dashi	1 cup	1	0
Miso	1 oz.	1	0

Satisfying Snacks

	Calories	Fat (g)	Fiber (g)
Crunchy Snacks			
Apple, 1 whole	81	0.5	2.8
Breadstick, 1 crisp	112	1.6	1.6
Broccoli, 1 cup raw flowerets	25	0.3	2.2
Carrot, 1 raw	31	0.1	2.3
Cauliflower, 1 cup flowerets	24	0.2	2.4
Celery, 1 stalk	6	0.1	0.6
Cracker, 1	23	0.8	0.6
Dill pickle, 1 large	24	0.3	2.1
Finn Crisp crackers, 4	76	0.8	1.8
Lahvosh Round, 1	28	0.1	0.2
Matzo cracker, 1	112	0.8	0.8
Melba rounds, 5	65	0.5	0.5
Oyster crackers, 24	72	2.4	0.6
Pear, 1 whole	98	0.7	4.3
Popcorn popped in oil, 3 cups	141	6.6	3.6
Popcorn, air popped, 3 cups	93	1.2	3.6
Rice cake, 1	34	0.3	0.5
Chewy Snacks			
Cheese pizza (thin crust), 1/8 medium pie	171	5.0	1.2
Dried apple, 4 slices	60	0.0	2.4
Dried apricots, 7 pieces	63	0.0	2.1
English muffin, wheat, 1 whole	145	3.2	2.5
Fig Newton, 1	56	0.9	0.7
Raisins, 2 tablespoons	58	0.2	1.0
Raisin Squares cereal (Kellogg's), 1/2 cup	90	0.0	2.0
Wheat bagel, 2 halves toasted	153	0.7	4.3
Savory or Salty Snacks			
Bean dip, 1/4 cup with raw veggies	82	2.8	2.0
Cheese, Lite Line or Weight Watchers, 1 oz.	54	2.3	0.0
Chicken, white meat canned, 1 ounce	47	2.3	0.0
Crab, 3 ounces	87	1.5	0.0
Ham, 95% lean, 1 ounce	41	1.6	0.0
Lean roast beef, 1 ounce	51	1.4	0.0
Mozzarella cheese, part skim, 1 ounce	79	4.9	0.0
Pretzels, 1 ounce	110	1.8	0.8
Taco sauce, 1/3 cup as a dip with raw veggies	32	0.0	0.6
Tuna, packed in water, 1 ounce	37	0.1	0.0
Turkey, white meat, no skin, 1 ounce	47	1.1	0.0

	Calories	Fat (g)	Fiber (g)
Sweet Snacks			
Angel food cake, all flavors, 1/12 cake	140	0.0	0.2
Banana, 9-inch, 1	105	0.6	2.2
Bing cherries, 12	60	1.2	1.2
Blueberries, 3/4 cup fresh	61	0.5	3.7
Bran flake cereal with raisins, 1 cup	174	1.1	7.6
Cone for ice cream, 1	41	0.3	0.4
Corn Bran cereal (Quaker), 1/2 cup	90	1.0	5.1
Frosted Mini Wheats (Kellogg's), 1 ounce	100	0.0	3.0
Graham crackers, 1 square	30	0.8	0.2
Grapes, 15	45	0.0	0.0
Hard candy, 1 piece	10	0.0	0.0
Jellied candy, 1 ounce	100	0.0	0.0
Jello gelatin, 1 cup	142	0.0	0.0
Kiwifruit, 1 medium	46	0.3	2.6
Licorice, 1 ounce	100	0.3	0.3
Melon, 1 cup chunks	99	0.5	2.3
Molasses cookie, 2-inch	48	1.8	0.2
Orange, 1 fresh	62	0.2	3.1
Peach, 1 fresh	37	0.1	1.4
Pineapple, 3/4 cup fresh			
or 1/2 cup canned in juice	57	0.5	1.4
Plums, 2 fresh	72	0.8	2.0
Strawberries, 1 cup fresh	45	0.6	3.9
Vanilla wafers, 6	102	4.8	0.2
Chocolate Snacks			
Cocoa Krispies, cereal, dry 1 ounce	110	0.0	0.8
Chocolate nonfat milk, 1 cup	140	0.4	1.3
Carnation Instant Breakfast, Chocolate Malt			
made with 1 cup skim milk	215	2.0	1.0
Chocolate pudding			
made with 1 cup skim milk,	129	0.8	0.5
Chocolate pudding pop, 1	80	2.0	0.0
Fudgesicle, 1 bar	98	0.2	1.0
Creamy or Frozen Snacks			
Applesauce,			
unsweetened with cinnamon, 1/2 cup	53	0.1	2.0
Cottage Cheese, 1% fat, 1/4 cup	41	0.6	0.0
Fruit and Creme Bar, 1	90	1.0	0.0
Fruit and juice bar, 1 (such as Dole)	70	0.0	0.0
Ice milk, 1/2 cup	92	2.8	0.0
Lemon frozen fruit bar, 1	50	0.0	0.0
Popsicle, 1	96	0.0	0.0

	Calories	Fat (g)	Fiber (g)
Pudding, made with skim milk, all flavors except chocolate, 1 cup	137	0.4	0.0
Sherbet, 1/2 cup	136	2.0	0.0
Sorbet, 1/2 cup	120	1.0	0.0
Yogurt, nonfat frozen, 1/2 cup	99	1.1	0.0
Yogurt, nonfat with fruit (Dannon Light), 1 cup	100	0.5	1.1
Thirst-Quenching Snacks			
Apple cider, 1/2 cup	59	0.0	0.0
Cranberry juice, 1/2 cup	72	0.1	0.0
Grapefruit juice, 1/2 cup	47	0.2	0.2
Lemonade, 1 cup	99	0.1	0.7
Orange or pineapple juice, 1/2 cup	56	0.1	0.4
Skim milk, 1 cup	86	0.4	0.0
V-8 Juice, 6 ounces	35	0.2	1.4
Warm Snacks			
Hot tomato juice, 6 ounces	30	0.2	1.4
Oatmeal, 1/2 cup	73	1.2	1.8
Tea or herbal tea, 1 cup	2	0.0	0.0
Vegetable bouillon, 1 packet	8	0.2	0.0
Vegetable beef or Chicken noodle soup, canned, 1 cup	83	3.1	0.5
Hot apple cider, 1 cup	117	0.3	0.0

Appendix B

Using Good Nutrition to Combat Cancer Treatment Side Effects

Table of Contents

Eating Well During Cancer Treatment

Your diet is an important part of your treatment for cancer. Eating the right kinds of foods during your treatment can help you feel better and stay stronger. The material contained in this index may also be useful after you finish treatment. Use it as a reference to be consulted any time that eating well is a challenge.

Your registered dietitian, doctor and nurse are your best sources of diet information. The material in this appendix will add to their advice. Feel free to ask them for help and to talk with them about changes in your diet. Ask them to explain or repeat anything that you do not understand.

A nutritious diet is always vital for your body to work at its best. Good nutrition is even more important for people with cancer. Why?

• Patients who eat well during their treatment are better able to cope with the side effects of treatment. They may even be able to handle a higher dose of certain treatments.
• A healthy diet can help keep up your strength, prevent the breakdown of body tissues and rebuild tissues damaged by cancer treatment.
• When you are unable to eat enough food or the right kind of food, your body uses stored nutrients as a source of energy. As a result, your natural defenses are weaker and your body cannot fight infection as well. Yet, this defense system is especially important to you now, because cancer patients are often at risk of getting infections.

It is important to eat a variety of foods every day. No one food or group of foods contains all of the nutrients you need. A diet to keep your body strong should include daily servings from these food groups:

Fruits and Vegetables Raw or cooked vegetables, fruits, and fruit juices provide vitamins, such as A and C, and minerals the body needs.

Protein Foods Protein helps your body heal itself and fight infection. Meat, fish, poultry, eggs and cheese give you protein as well as many vitamins and minerals.

Grains Bread, pasta and cereals provide a variety of carbohydrates and B vitamins. Carbohydrates are a good source of energy, which the body needs to function well.

Dairy Foods Milk and other dairy products provide protein and many vitamins and are the best source of calcium.

The chart on page 181, "Eat a Variety of Foods Each Day," shows recommended guidelines for a healthful diet. While these standards are a good goal, you also need to listen to your body. If you get nauseous eating fruits but can keep protein foods down, feel free to eat more protein and less fruit. Anything you eat will be a plus in helping you get enough calories and maintain your weight.

The NCI recommends that you ask your doctor or nutritionist before taking any vitamin or mineral supplements. Too much of some vitamins or minerals can be just as dangerous as too little. Large doses of some vitamins may even stop your cancer treatment from working the way it should. To avoid problems, don't take these products on your own. Always follow your doctor's instructions.

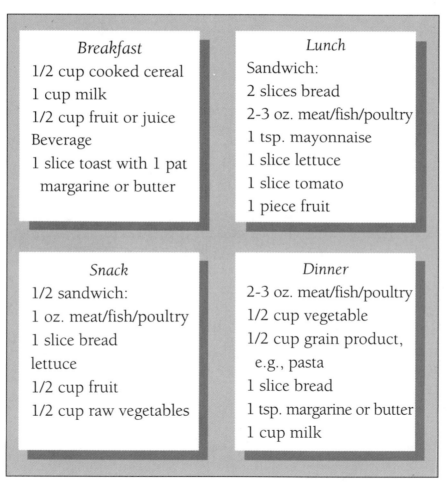

Breakfast
1/2 cup cooked cereal
1 cup milk
1/2 cup fruit or juice
Beverage
1 slice toast with 1 pat
   margarine or butter

Lunch
Sandwich:
2 slices bread
2-3 oz. meat/fish/poultry
1 tsp. mayonnaise
1 slice lettuce
1 slice tomato
1 piece fruit

Snack
1/2 sandwich:
1 oz. meat/fish/poultry
1 slice bread
lettuce
1/2 cup fruit
1/2 cup raw vegetables

Dinner
2-3 oz. meat/fish/poultry
1/2 cup vegetable
1/2 cup grain product,
   e.g., pasta
1 slice bread
1 tsp. margarine or butter
1 cup milk

SAMPLE MENU, INCLUDING MINIMUM NUMBER OF SERVINGS FROM EACH FOOD GROUP

EAT A VARIETY OF FOODS EACH DAY

Food Group	Suggested Daily Servings	What Counts as a Serving?
Breads, Cereals, and other Grain Products Whole-grain enriched	6 servings from entire group (include several servings of whole-grain products daily.)	1 slice of bread 1/2 hamburger bun or English muffin 1 small roll, biscuit or muffin 3 to 4 small or 2 large crackers 1/2 cup cooked cereal, rice or pasta, 1 oz. ready-to-eat breakfast cereal
Fats, Sweets, and Alcoholic Beverages	Avoid fats and sweets. If you drink alcoholic beverages, do so in moderation.	
Fruits Citrus, melon, berries Other fruits	2 servings from entire group	1 whole fruit such as medium apple, banana, or orange 1/2 grapefruit 1 melon wedge 3/4 cup juice 1/2 cup berries 1/2 cup cooked or canned fruit 1/4 cup dried fruit
Vegetables Dark-green leafy Deep-yellow Dry beans and peas (legumes) Starchy Other vegetables	3 servings from entire group. Include all types regularly. Use dark-green leafy vegetables and dry beans and peas several times a week.	1/2 cup cooked or chopped raw vegetables 1 cup leafy raw vegetables, such as lettuce or spinach

Food Group	Suggested Daily Servings	What Counts as a Serving?
Meat, Poultry, Fish and Alternates (eggs, dry beans and peas, nuts and seeds)	2 servings from entire group	Amounts should total 5 to 7 oz. of cooked lean meat, poultry or fish a day. Count 1 egg, 1/2 cup cooked beans or 2 tbsp. peanut butter as 1 oz. of meat.
Milk, Cheese and Yogurt	2 servings from entire group. 3 servings for women who are pregnant or breast-feeding; 4 servings for teens who are pregnant or breast-feeding.	1 cup milk 8 oz. yogurt 1½ oz. natural cheese 2 oz. processed cheese

Source: USDA "Preparing Foods and Planning Menus using The Dietary Guidelines."

Coping With Side Effects During Treatment

All the usual methods of treating cancer—surgery, radiation therapy, chemotherapy and biological therapy—have to be very powerful to be effective. Although treatments target the cancer cells in your body, they unavoidably damage normal, healthy cells at the same time. This often produces unpleasant side effects that cause eating problems (See chart, page 184.)

Cancer treatment side effects of vary from patient to patient. The part of the body being treated, length of treatment and the dose of treatment also affect whether side effects will occur. Ask your doctor about how your treatment may affect you.

The good news is that only about one-third of cancer patients have side effects during treatment. Most side effects go away when treatment ends. Your doctor will try to plan a treatment that keeps side effects down.

Cancer treatment may also affect your eating in another way. People who are upset, worried or afraid may have eating problems. Losing your appetite and experiencing nausea are two normal responses to feeling nervous or fearful. Such problems should last a short time.

While you are in the hospital, your health-care team can help you plan your diet. They can also help you solve your physical or emotional eating problems. Feel free to talk to them if problems arise during your recovery as well. Ask them what has worked for their other patients.

Don't be afraid to give food a chance. Not everyone has problems with eating during cancer treatment. Even those who experience eating problems have days when eating is a pleasure.

This section offers practical hints for coping with treatment side effects that may affect your eating. These suggestions have helped other patients manage eating problems that can be frustrating to handle. Try all the ideas to find what works best for you. Share your needs and concerns with your family and friends, particularly those who prepare meals for you. Let them know that you appreciate their support as you work to take control of eating problems.

HOW CANCER TREATMENTS CAN AFFECT EATING

Effects On Body	Effects On Eating

Surgery

Increases the need for good nutrition by putting stress on the body. Parts of the body needed for eating, such as stomach, mouth and throat may not work properly. Treatment may also make them sore.

Before surgery, a high-protein, high-calorie diet may be prescribed if a patient is under-weight or weak. After surgery, some patients may not resume normal eating at first. They may receive nutrients:
Through a needle in their vein (IV or intravenous feeding)
Through a tube in their nose or stomach
By drinking clear liquids
By following a full-liquid diet

Radiation Therapy

May harm parts of the body as it damages cancer cells.

Treatment of head, neck or chest may cause:
Dry mouth
Sore mouth
Sore throat
Change in taste of food
Dental problems
Treatment of stomach may cause:
Nausea
Vomiting
Diarrhea

Chemotherapy

May harm parts of the body needed for eating as it destroys cancer cells.

Nausea and vomiting
Loss of appetite
Diarrhea
Constipation
Sore mouth or throat
Weight gain
Change in taste of food

Biological Therapy (Immunotherapy)

Not known

Nausea and vomiting
Diarrhea
Sore mouth
Severe weight loss (anorexia)
Dry mouth.
Change in taste of food.

Loss of Appetite

Loss of appetite or poor appetite is one of the most common problems that occur with cancer and its treatment. Many things affect appetite, including feeling sick (having nausea, vomiting) and being upset or depressed about having cancer. A person who has these feelings, whether physical or emotional, may not be interested in eating.

You may find the following suggestions helpful in making mealtimes more enjoyable and making yourself feel more like eating:

- Stay calm, especially at mealtime. Don't hurry your meals.
- Involve yourself in as many normal activities as possible. But, if you feel uneasy and do not want to take part, don't force yourself.
- Try changing the time, place and surroundings of meals. A candlelight dinner can make mealtime more appealing. Set a colorful table. Listen to soft music while eating. Eat with others or watch your favorite TV program while you eat.
- Eat whenever you are hungry. Several smaller meals throughout the day may be even better than three large meals.
- Eat a variety of foods often during the day, even at bedtime. Have healthy snacks handy. Taking just a few bites of the right foods or sips of the right liquids every hour or so can help you get more protein and calories.

Sore Mouth or Throat

Mouth sores, tender gums and a sore throat or esophagus often result from radiation therapy, anticancer drugs and infection. If you have a sore mouth or gums, see your doctor to be sure the soreness is a treatment side effect and not an unrelated dental problem. The doctor may be able to give you medicine that will control mouth and throat pain. Your dentist also can give you tips for care of your mouth.

Certain foods will irritate an already tender mouth and make chewing and swallowing difficult. By carefully choosing the foods you eat and by taking good care of your mouth, you can usually make eating easier. Some suggestions that may help include:

- Try soft foods that are easy to chew and swallow such as:
  Milkshakes
  Bananas, applesauce and other soft fruits
  Peach, pear and apricot nectars
  Watermelon
  Cottage cheese
  Mashed potatoes, macaroni and cheese
  Custards, puddings and gelatin
  Scrambled eggs
  Oatmeal or other cooked cereals
  Puréed or mashed vegetables such as peas and
    carrots
  Puréed meats
  Liquids

• Cook foods slowly and for long periods until they are soft and tender.
• Cut foods into small pieces.
• Mix food with butter, thin gravies and sauces to make it easier to swallow.
• Use a blender or food processor to purée your food.
• Use a straw to drink liquids.
• Try foods cold or at room temperature. Hot or warm foods can irritate a tender mouth and throat.
• Avoid foods that can irritate your mouth, such as:
    Citrus fruit or juice such as oranges, grapefruits and tangerines.
    Spicy or salty foods.
    Rough, coarse or dry foods such as raw vegetables, granola and toast.
• If swallowing is hard, tilting your head back or moving it forward may help.
• If your teeth and gums are sore, your dentist may be able to recommend a special product for cleaning your teeth.
• Rinse your mouth with water often to remove food and bacteria and to promote healing.
• Ask your doctor about anesthetic lozenges and sprays that can numb the mouth and throat long enough for you to eat meals.

Changed Sense of Taste

Your sense of taste may change. Chemotherapy, radiation therapy or the cancer itself may cause this to occur. Sometimes called *mouth blindness* or *taste blindness*, it may cause a change in the way foods taste. Some patients complain of a bitter, metallic taste, especially when eating meat or other protein foods. Patients also may find that many foods have less taste. This is usually a short-term problem.

Each person's taste may be affected differently. You will need to learn which, if any, foods taste different to you. Depending on how your taste has been affected, some of the following ideas for improving flavor may work better than others. In addition, visit your dentist to check for dental problems that may affect taste. Also ask your dentist about special mouthwashes and good mouth care.

Here are tips to help your food taste better.

- Choose and prepare foods that look and smell good to you.
- If red meat (such as beef) tastes strange, substitute chicken, turkey, eggs, dairy products or fish that doesn't have a strong smell.
- Help the flavor of meat, chicken or fish by marinating it in sweet fruit juices, sweet wine, Italian dressing or sweet and sour sauce.
- Try using small amounts of flavorful seasonings such as basil, oregano or rosemary.
- Try tart foods such as oranges or lemonade that may have more taste. A tart lemon custard might taste good

and will also provide needed protein and calories. Do not try this if you have a sore mouth or throat.

- Serve foods at room temperature.
- Try using bacon, ham, or onion to add flavor to vegetables.
- Stop eating foods that cause an unpleasant taste.

Nausea

Nausea, with or without vomiting, is a common side effect of surgery, chemotherapy, radiation therapy and immunotherapy. The disease itself, or other conditions unrelated to your cancer or treatment, may also cause nausea. Whatever the cause, nausea can keep you from getting enough food and needed nutrients. Here are some ideas that may be helpful.

- Ask your doctor about medicine to help control nausea.
- Try foods such as:
  Toast and crackers
  Yogurt
  Sherbet
  Pretzels
  Angel food cake
  Oatmeal
  Skinned chicken—prepare baked or broiled, not fried
  Soft or bland fruits and vegetables, such as canned peaches
  Clear liquids, sipped slowly
  Ice chips

- Avoid foods such as:

    Fatty, greasy or fried foods

    Very sweet foods such as candy, cookies or cake

    Spicy, hot foods

    Foods with strong odors

- Eat small amounts often and slowly.
- Avoid eating in a room that's stuffy or too warm, or one with cooking odors or smells that might disagree with you.
- Drink fewer liquids with meals. Drinking liquids can cause a full, bloated feeling.
- Drink or sip liquids throughout the day, except at mealtimes. Using a straw may help.
- Drink beverages that are cool or chilled. Try freezing favorite beverages in ice-cube trays.
- Eat foods at room temperature or cooler. Hot foods may add to nausea.
- Don't force yourself to eat favorite foods when you feel nauseated. This may cause a permanent dislike of those foods.
- Rest after meals, because activity may slow digestion. It's best to rest sitting up for about an hour after meals.
- If nausea is a problem in the morning, try eating dry toast or crackers before getting up.
- Wear loose-fitting clothes.
- Avoid eating for one to two hours before treatment if nausea occurs during radiation therapy or chemotherapy.

•Try to keep track of when your nausea occurs and what causes it. It could be specific foods, events or surroundings. If possible, make appropriate changes in your diet or schedule. Share this information with your doctor or nurse.

Vomiting

Vomiting may follow nausea and may be brought on by treatment, food odors, gas in the stomach or bowel or motion. In some people, certain surroundings, such as the hospital, may cause vomiting.

If vomiting is severe or lasts for more than a few days, contact your doctor.

Often, if you can control nausea, you can prevent vomiting. At times, however, you may not be able to prevent either nausea or vomiting. You may find some relief by using relaxation exercises or meditation. These usually involve deep rhythmic breathing and quiet concentration. Such exercises can be done almost anywhere. If vomiting occurs, try these hints to prevent further episodes:

•Ask your doctor about medicine to control nausea.
•Do not drink or eat until you have the vomiting under control.
•Once you have controlled vomiting, try small amounts of clear liquids. Begin with a teaspoonful every 10 minutes. Gradually increase the amount to a tablespoonful every 20 minutes. Finally, try 2 tablespoonfuls every 30 minutes.

•When you are able to keep down clear liquids, try a full liquid diet. Continue taking small amounts as often as you can keep them down. Gradually work up to your regular diet.

Diarrhea

Diarrhea can be caused by several things, including chemotherapy, radiation therapy to the abdomen, infection, food sensitivity and emotional upset.

Long-term or severe diarrhea may cause other problems. During diarrhea food passes quickly through the bowel—before the body can absorb vitamins, minerals and water. This may cause dehydration, when your body doesn't have enough water. It may also increase the risk of infection. Contact your doctor if the diarrhea is severe or lasts for more than a couple of days. Here are some ideas for coping with diarrhea:

•Try these nutritious low-fiber foods:
   Yogurt
   Rice or noodles
   Grape juice
   Farina or cream of wheat
   Eggs (cooked until the whites are solid, not fried)
   Ripe bananas
   Puréed vegetables
   Canned or cooked fruit without skins, such as
      applesauce
   Smooth peanut butter

White bread

Chicken or turkey, skinned

Tender or ground beef

Fish

Cottage cheese, cream cheese

- Avoid eating foods such as:

  Greasy, fatty or fried foods

  Raw vegetables and fruits

  High-fiber vegetables such as broccoli, corn, beans, cabbage, peas and cauliflower

  Strong spices, such as hot pepper, curry and Cajun spice mix

- Eat small amounts of food and liquids throughout the day instead of three large meals.

- Drink plenty of liquids during the day. Drinking fluids is important because your body may not get enough water when you have diarrhea.

- Drink liquids that are at room temperature. Avoid very hot or very cold foods.

- Eat plenty of foods and liquids that contain sodium (salt) and potassium. These minerals are often lost during diarrhea. Good choices for liquids include bouillon or fat-free broth. Foods high in potassium that don't cause diarrhea include bananas, peach and apricot nectar, and boiled or mashed potatoes.

- After sudden short-term attacks of diarrhea (acute diarrhea), try a clear liquid diet during the first 12 to 14 hours. This lets the bowel rest while replacing important body fluids lost during diarrhea.

- Limit foods and beverages that contain caffeine. These include coffee, strong tea, some soft drinks and chocolate.
- Use milk and milk products with caution. Diarrhea may be caused by lactose intolerance, an inability to digest the lactose in milk. See page 195.

Constipation

Some anticancer drugs and other drugs such as pain medicines may cause constipation. This problem also may occur if your diet lacks enough fluid or bulk, or if you have been bedridden. Here are some suggestions to prevent and treat constipation:

- Drink plenty of liquids. This will help keep stools soft.
- Take a hot drink about one-half hour before your usual time for a bowel movement.
- Eat high-fiber foods such as whole grains, and raw fresh vegetables and fruits such as cauliflower, potatoes with skin, peas, bananas, pears, oranges and berries.
- Get some exercise every day. Taking a brisk walk is excellent. Talk to your doctor or a physical therapist about the amount and type of exercise that is right for you.
- Add unprocessed wheat bran to foods such as casseroles and homemade breads.

•If none of these suggestions work, ask your doctor about medicine to ease constipation. Check with your doctor before taking any laxatives or stool softeners.

Weight Gain

Sometimes patients gain excess weight during treatment without eating extra calories. Certain anticancer drugs, such as *prednisone*, can cause the body to retain fluid so patients gain weight. The extra weight is in the form of water and does not mean you are eating too much.

Do not go on a diet if you notice weight gain. Instead, tell your doctor so you can find out what may be causing this change. If anticancer drugs are causing weight gain, the doctor may recommend limiting the salt you eat—salt causes your body to retain water. Drugs called *diuretics* also may be prescribed to get rid of extra fluid.

Lactose Intolerance

Lactose intolerance means that your body can't digest or absorb the milk sugar called *lactose*. Milk, other dairy products and foods to which milk has been added contain lactose.

Lactose intolerance may occur after treatment with some antibiotics or with radiation to the stomach or any treatment that affects the digestive tract. The part of your intestines that breaks down lactose may not work properly during treatment. For some people the symptoms—gas, cramping and diarrhea—disappear a few weeks or months after the treatments end or when the intestine heals. For those who continue to experience lactose intolerance, a permanent change in eating habits may be required.

If you have this problem, your doctor may advise you to follow a diet low in foods that contain lactose. If milk had been a main source of protein in your diet, it will be important to get enough protein from other foods. Products such as soybean formulas and aged cheeses are good sources of protein and other nutrients.

Your body may be able to deal with milk that has been treated with *acidophilus* bacteria, sometimes labled *Sweet-A* milk. There are also tablets that can be added to milk to change the lactose structure so the milk can be digested.

Saving Time and Energy

Your body needs both rest and nourishment during and after treatment for cancer. If you are usually the cook, here are some suggestions for saving time and energy in preparing meals.

- Let someone else do the cooking when possible.
- If you know that your recovery time from treatment or surgery is going to be longer than one or two days, prepare a helper list. Decide who can help you shop, cook, set the table and clean up. Write it down, discuss it and post it where it can easily be seen. If children help, give them a small reward.
- Write out menus, choosing things that you or your family can prepare easily. Casseroles, TV dinners,

hot dogs, hamburgers and meals that you have prepared and frozen ahead are good ideas. Cook larger
batches to be frozen so you will have them for
future use. Add instructions so other people can
help you.

•Use shopping lists. Keep them handy so that they can
be used as guides either by you or by other people.

•When making casseroles for freezing, partially cook rice
and macaroni products. They will cook further in the
reheating process. Add 1/2 cup liquid to refrigerated
or frozen casseroles when reheating because they often
dry out during refrigeration. Frozen casseroles take a
long time to heat completely—at least 45 minutes in
deep dishes in the oven. Reheating in the microwave
is much faster, but be sure to reposition (turn) the
casserole occasionally to ensure even heating.

•Don't be shy about accepting gifts of food and offers
of help from family and friends. Let them know
what you like and offer your recipes. If people bring
food you can't use right away, freeze it. That home-
cooked meal can break the monotony of quickie
suppers. It can also save time when you're on a tight
schedule. Date the food when you put it in the
refrigerator or freezer.

•Have as few dishes, pots and pans to wash as possible. Soak dirty dishes to cut down washing time.
Cook in dishes and pans that can double as serving
dishes. Use paper napkins and disposable plates,
especially for desserts. Paper cups are fine for kids

and for taking liquid medicines. Disposable pans are great timesavers. Foil containers from frozen foods work well.

•When you are preparing soft dishes, choose foods the whole family can eat. Omelets, scrambled eggs, macaroni and cheese, meat loaf, tuna-salad sand-wiches and tuna casseroles are good choices. Set aside enough food to be puréed in the blender or food processor for yourself.

•Use mixes, frozen ready-to-eat main dishes and take-out foods whenever possible. The less time spent cooking and cleaning up, the more time for relax-ation and the family.

•If someone is cooking for you, share this information with them for ideas for food selection and prepara-tion. They will also get a better sense of your special needs.

Adapted from: "Eating Hints—Recipes & Tips for Better Nutrition During Cancer Treatment" (National Cancer Institute Publication #92-2079)

Appendix C

Current Research & New Theories

Table of Contents

Genes-Colon-Cancer Connection

A medical study announced in May 1993 described the discovery of a gene that could be a source of colon cancer. It is estimated that the gene is found in about 1 out of 200 people. It possibly causes one in seven instances of colon cancer, according to Dr. Bert Volgelstein of Johns Hopkins Oncology Center.

It is estimated 70% to 90% of the people who have the gene will get some form of cancer. If cancer does not develop in the colon, it could be found in the uterus, ovary, stomach, small intestine, gall bladder, pancreas or kidney. About half the women who have this gene and who do not develop colon cancer can be expected to develop uterine cancer.

The announcement of a medical breakthrough is just the first step on the long road to finding a treatment. Independent study is always undertaken to seek evidence supporting or contradicting the new theory. Yet, respected researchers from a few of the world's leading medical institutions, including the University of Helsinki, Johns Hopkins University and the Mayo Clinic, provide great credibility for this particular research effort.

As scientific study continues, the next step will be to develop a test to find the 1 in 200 people with the gene. Because it is thought to be inherited, the first genetic tests will be directed to high-risk people with family histories of colorectal cancer. Screening procedures may then be extended to average-risk people in the general population. Identifying people with the gene, when cancer is in the start-up stages, should lead to earlier cures and lower mortality rates.

Researchers at Memorial Sloan-Kettering Cancer Center are also focusing on a gene-cancer connection. They have identified specific gene mutations that appear to lead to colorectal cancer. In the future this type of information may help doctors know which type of treatment will work best for each individual patient.

Impact of Aspirin

In the late 1940s, California general practitioner Lawrence Craven began advising his patients to take two aspirins a day. Thereafter, he became fascinated when he discovered the fast flow of blood during tonsillectomies performed on his patients who took aspirin. Realizing that aspirin could possibly help prevent blood clotting, he began to chronicle the health of thousands of aspirin-taking men. In 1956, he reported that there were no heart attacks among the patients who took aspirin.

Over 40 years later, medical experts are gradually giving more support to aspirin's capabilities in combating a wide range of diseases, including cancer, heart disease, cataracts, Alzheimer's and AIDS. Two different 1991 studies completed by the American Cancer Society and a Boston University team showed that regular use of aspirin, or aspirin-containing drugs (called *NSAIDs*, for non-steroidal anti-inflammatory drugs) may cut the risk of dying from colorectal cancer in half. In addition, some researchers believe aspirin may help prevent the development of colorectal cancer.

More recently, Dr. Edward Giovanucci of the Harvard Medical School announced the results of another study originally designed to evaluate general health problems. In 1986, 1988 and 1990, approximately 48,000 male health professionals completed questionnaires. The results indicated taking aspirin two or more times a week resulted in 32% less chance of having colorectal cancer and cut in half the risk of developing metastatic colorectal cancer, cancer that has spread.

Dr. Garret Fitzgerald is a professor of cardiovascular

medicine at the University of Pennsylvania, and one of the world's foremost experts on aspirin. Dr. Fitzgerald observed that "no little white pill does everything, that's for sure. But the strength of the evidence for aspirin working where it has been shown to work is probably greater than the strength of evidence for any drug for human disease."

There is still much disagreement as to the value of aspirin in preventing colorectal cancer as well as other illnesses. There is also concern about aspirin's possible side effects, such as the development of colitis, ulcers and diverticular disease. Complications may also be caused by thinning of the blood that can result from regular long-term aspirin intake. Many different studies are now underway. Perhaps they can provide more definitive answers in the future.

Calcium

Various studies during the past ten years have produced conflicting results regarding the role of calcium in preventing colorectal cancer. What was considered by some to be a plausible theory in the mid-1980s seems to have lost most of its supporters in the 1990s. Research on the subject is continuing. Currently, it is recommended that adults should have daily calcium intake of about 800mg per day as a way of promoting general good health.

Garlic

It has been known for some time that eating garlic may lower a person's risk of developing colon cancer. Recent research at

Pennsylvania State University has shown that a chemical found in garlic may actually help shrink tumors. This could lead to a role for garlic in treating cancer.

Smoking

Several preliminary studies indicate a link between long-term smoking and colorectal cancer. The speculation centers around cancer-causing compounds released by cigarettes that could reach the large bowel through the circulatory or digestive systems.

Folic Acid

According to a recent study, heavy drinkers are more vulnerable to colon cancer than light drinkers, but this can be counteracted by eating foods high in folic acid. It appears that folic acid helps to suppress the activation of cancer-causing genes. The primary sources of folic acid are green vegetables, fresh fruits, liver and yeast.

It was determined that the amount of folic acid needed was about 650 milligrams per day. This is the equivalent of one cup of cooked lentils, one cup of cooked spinach and an orange. Folic acid may also be taken as a vitamin supplement.

Bile Acid

Bile is a greenish-yellow fluid used by the body to digest fats. It is produced in the liver, stored in the gall bladder and released into the small bowel. The more fat you eat, the more bile acid is produced. There is some laboratory evidence that excess bile acids may cause cancerous changes in the cells lining the large bowel.

Phytochemicals

In addition to being good sources of fiber, fruits and vegetables contain a variety of compounds that appear to have cancer-prevention properties. These compounds are called *phytochemicals*. ("Phyto" comes from a Greek word meaning "plant.") There are literally thousands of phytochemicals in plants. Phytochemicals help fruits and vegetables to grow and thrive. Studies show that they may have a beneficial effect on humans as well.

Phytochemicals may work in a number of ways to block the effects of cancer-causing agents. The body has many natural, built-in mechanisms to combat harmful substances that enter the body. Scientists believe that some phytochemicals increase the level and functioning of these protective mechanisms, thus enhancing the body's natural ability to prevent cancer.

Research into phytochemicals is now at the beginning stages. What can be said is that current knowledge supports the idea that fruits and vegetables are good for your health. There is no evidence that phytochemicals are found in vitamin pills.

Estrogen Therapy

A study reported in the Journal of the National Cancer Institute on April 5, 1995, suggests that women who take estrogen to alleviate symptoms of menopause may also lower their risk of colon and rectal cancer. After adjusting for other factors, such as body weight, parental history and race, researchers found a significantly lower death rate from colon cancer among women who had taken estrogen at some point in their lives. Those who had used the treatment for more than 10 years cut their risk by nearly half. The results were similar for rectal cancer.

Further research is necessary, particularly since the current study was based on cancer deaths and not the incidence of new cases.

Detection Technology

Dr. David J. Vining of Wake Forest University in New Orleans is the principal developer of a tubeless colon exam. Called *virtual colonoscopy*, it combines X-ray and computer technology to provide a 3-D, from-the-inside view of the colon. The X-ray machine spins around the patient, taking 400 to 500 pictures in half a minute. The doctor guides the X-ray equipment and watches the changing pictures on a computer screen. Vining estimates that the exam will cost $450 to $650, much less than a colonoscopy.

Questions regarding accuracy have not been answered. For example, how many tumors can be expected to be missed by the test? And how many non-tumors will be wrongly interpreted as tumors?

The virtual colonoscopy could be a valuable detection procedure—it is not yet a replacement for the colonoscopy. Once such a procedure indicates the presence of a mysterious growth in the large bowel a colonoscopy will be performed to cut out the growth or take a biopsy.

Appendix D

American Cancer Society Divisions

National Headquarters: American Cancer Society, Inc.
1599 Clifton Road N.E., Atlanta, GA 30329-4251
Phone 1-800-ACS-2345 (1-800-227-2345)

Alabama Division, Inc.
504 Brookwood Boulevard
Homewood, AL 35209
(205) 879-2242

Alaska Division, Inc.
406 West Fireweed Lane
Anchorage, AK 99503
(907) 277-8696

Arizona Division, Inc.
2929 East Thomas Road
Phoenix, AZ 85016
(602) 224-0524

Arkansas Division, Inc.
901 North University
Little Rock, AR 72203
(501) 664-3480

California Division, Inc.
1710 Webster Street
Oakland, CA 94612
(510) 893-7900

Colorado Division, Inc.
2255 South Oneida
Denver, CO 80224
(303) 758-2030

Connecticut Division, Inc.
Barnes Park South
14 Village Lane
Wallingford, CT 06492
(203) 265-7161

Delaware Division, Inc.
92 Read's Way
New Castle, DE 19720
(302) 324-4227

District of Columbia Division, Inc.
1875 Connecticut Avenue, N.W.
Washington, DC 20009
(202) 483-2600

Florida Division, Inc.
3709 West Jetton Avenue
Tampa, FL 33629-5146
(813) 253-0541

Georgia Division, Inc.
2200 Lake Boulevard
Atlanta, GA 30319
(404) 816-7800

Hawaii Pacific Division, Inc.
Community Services Center Bldg.
200 North Vineyard Boulevard
Honolulu, HI 96817
(808) 531-1662

Idaho Division, Inc.
2676 Vista Avenue
Boise, ID 83705-0836
(208) 343-4609

Illinois Division, Inc.
77 East Monroe
Chicago, IL 60603-5795
(312) 641-6150

Indiana Division, Inc.
8730 Commerce Park Place
Indianapolis, IN 46268
(317) 872-4432

Iowa Division, Inc.
8364 Hickman Road
Des Moines, IA 50325
(515) 253-0147

Kansas Division, Inc.
1315 S.W. Arrowhead Road
Topeka, KS 66604
(913) 273-4114

Kentucky Division, Inc.
701 West Muhammed Ali Blvd.
Louisville, KY 40203-1909
(502) 584-6782

Louisiana Division, Inc.
2200 Veteran's Memorial Blvd.
Suite 214
Kenner, LA 70062
(504) 469-0021

Maine Division, Inc.
52 Federal Street
Brunswick, ME 04011
(207) 729-3339

Maryland Division, Inc.
8219 Town Center Drive
Baltimore, MD 21236-0026
(410) 931-6868

Massachusetts Division, Inc.
247 Commonwealth Avenue
Boston, MA 02116
(617) 267-2650

Michigan Division, Inc.
1205 East Saginaw Street
Lansing, MI 48906
(517) 371-2920

Minnesota Division, Inc.
3316 West 66th Street
Minneapolis, MN 55435
(612) 925-2772

Mississippi Division, Inc.
1380 Livingston Lane
Lakeover Office Park
Jackson, MS 39213
(601) 362-8874

Missouri Division, Inc.
3322 American Avenue
Jefferson City, MO 65102
(314) 893-4800

Montana Division, Inc.
17 North 26th
Billings, MT 59101
(406) 252-7111

Nebraska Division, Inc.
8502 West Center Road
Omaha, NE 68124-5255
(402) 393-5800

Nevada Division, Inc.
1325 East Harmon
Las Vegas, NV 89119
(702) 798-6857

New Hampshire Division, Inc.
360 Route 101, Unit 501
Bedford, NH 03110-5032
(603) 472-8899

New Jersey Division, Inc.
2600 US Highway 1
North Brunswick, NJ 08902-0803
(908) 297-8000

New Mexico Division, Inc.
5800 Lomas Boulevard, N.E.
Albuquerque, NM 87110
(505) 260-2105

New York State Division, Inc.
6725 Lyons Street
East Syracuse, NY 13057
(315) 437-7025

Long Island Division, Inc.
75 Davids Drive
Hauppauge, NY 11788
(516) 436-7070

New York City Division, Inc.
19 West 56th Street
New York, NY 10019
(212) 586-8700

Queens Division, Inc.
112-25 Queens Boulevard
Forest Hills, NY 11375
(718) 263-2224

Westchester Division, Inc.
30 Glenn Street
White Plains, NY 10603
(914) 949-4800

North Carolina Division, Inc.
11 South Boylan Avenue
Raleigh, NC 27603
(919) 834-8463

North Dakota Division, Inc.
123 Roberts Street
Fargo, ND 58102
(701) 232-1385

Ohio Division, Inc.
5555 Frantz Road
Dublin, OH 43017
(614) 889-9565

Oklahoma Division, Inc.
4323 63rd, Suite 110
Oklahoma City, OK 73116
(405) 843-9888

Oregon Division, Inc.
0330 S.W. Curry
Portland, OR 97201
(503) 295-6422

Pennsylvania Division, Inc.
Route 422 & Snipe Avenue
Hershey, PA 17033-0897
(717) 533-6144

Philadelphia Division, Inc.
1422 Chestnut Street
Philadelphia, PA 19102
(215) 665-2900

Puerto Rico Division, Inc.
Calle Alverio #577
Esquina Sargento Medina
Hato Rey, PR 00918
(809) 764-2295

Rhode Island Division, Inc.
400 Main Street
Pawtucket, RI 02860
(401) 722-8480

South Carolina Division, Inc.
128 Stonemark Lane
Columbia, SC 29210-3855
(803) 750-1693

South Dakota Division, Inc.
4101 Carnegie Place
Sioux Falls, SD 57106-2322
(605) 361-8277

Tennessee Division, Inc.
1315 Eighth Avenue, South
Nashville, TN 37203
(615) 255-1227

Texas Division, Inc.
2433 Ridgepoint Drive
Austin, TX 78754
(512) 928-2262

Utah Division, Inc.
941 East 3300 S.
Salt Lake City, UT 84106
(801) 483-1500

Vermont Division, Inc.
13 Loomis Street
Montpelier, VT 05602
(802) 223-2348

Virginia Division, Inc.
P.O. Box 6359
Glen Allen, VA 23058-6359
(804) 527-3700

Washington Division, Inc.
2120 First Avenue North
Seattle, WA 98109-1140
(206) 283-1152

West Virginia Division, Inc.
2428 Kanawha Boulevard East
Charleston, WV 25311
(304) 344-3611

Wisconsin Division, Inc.
P.O. Box 902
Pewaukee, WI 53072-0902
(414) 523-5500

Wyoming Division, Inc.
2222 House Avenue
Cheyenne, WY 82001
(307) 638-3331

Appendix E

NCI Community Clinical Oncology Program

The Community Clinical Oncology Program (CCOP) was established by the National Cancer Institute (NCI) in 1983. Through this program, community physicians work with scientists in conducting NCI-supported clinical trials. Clinical trials are research studies conducted with patients or with healthy people. They are designed to answer specific questions about the effectiveness of new ways to prevent, detect, diagnose and treat cancer.

Participation in the CCOP benefits patients and physicians in the community and scientists in research centers. The program helps in the transfer of the latest research findings to the community level. The CCOP increases the number of patients and physicians who can participate in clinical trials operated at major research centers. It allows scientists to conduct large-scale cancer-prevention and control studies.

Facilities participating in the CCOP are required to affiliate with at least one research base. A research base may be an NCI-supported clinical cooperative group or cancer center.

The CCOP participants use research protocols developed and provided by the research bases. They also enter patients into NCI-approved clinical trials through the research base(s) with which they are affiliated.

To obtain information about the CCOP in your area, call the Cancer Information Service at 1-800-4-CANCER (1-800-422-6237).

Appendix F

NCI Cancer Centers Program

The National Cancer Institute (NCI) Cancer Centers Program comprises more than 50 NCI-designated cancer centers engaged in multidisciplinary research efforts. Their goals are to reduce cancer incidence, morbidity and mortality.

Although some cancer centers existed in the late 1960s and 1970s, it was the National Cancer Act of 1971 that authorized the establishment of 15 new cancer centers, as well as continuing support for existing ones. This act dramatically transformed the centers' structure and broadened the scope of their mission to include all aspects of basic, clinical and cancer-control research. Since then the centers program has continued to grow and now includes four types of centers

Comprehensive cancer centers which emphasize a multidisciplinary approach to cancer research, patient care and community outreach. To attain recognition from NCI as a comprehensive cancer center, an institution must pass rigorous peer review. Under guidelines established in 1990, the criteria for comprehensiveness include:

- strong core of laboratory research in several fields, such as biology and molecular genetics;
- strong program of clinical research;
- ability to transfer research findings into clinical practice;
- strong participation in NCI-designated, high-priority clinical trials;
- significant levels of cancer-prevention and control research;
- important outreach and educational activities.

Three other types of cancer centers have special characteristics and capabilities for organizing new programs of research. They are intended to exploit important new findings or address timely research questions.

- Basic science cancer centers engage almost entirely in basic research. Some centers engage in collaborative research with outside clinical investigators and in cooperative projects with industry to generate medical applications from new discoveries in the laboratory.
- Clinical cancer centers focus on both basic and clinical research within the same institutional framework. They frequently incorporate nearby affiliated clinical-research institutions into their overall research programs.
- Consortium cancer centers concentrate on clinical research and cancer-prevention-and-control research. These centers work with state and local public health departments to transfer effective prevention-and-control techniques from their research findings to those institutions responsible for implementing population-wide public-health programs. Consortium centers also collaborate with institutions that conduct clinical-trial research and coordinate networks of community hospitals cooperating in clinical trials.

Together, NCI-designated cancer centers work toward discovering new and innovative approaches to cancer research and, through interdisciplinary efforts, to move this research from the laboratory into clinical trials and into clinical practice.

Following are addresses of the NCI-designated cancer centers. Information about referral procedures, treatment costs and services available to patients can be obtained from the individual cancer centers.

Comprehensive,* Clinical,** and Consortium Cancer Centers Supported by the National Cancer Institute

ALABAMA
University of Alabama at Birmingham
    Comprehensive Cancer Center*
Basic Health Sciences Building,
    Room 108
1918 University Boulevard
Birmingham, AL 35294
(205) 934-5077

ARIZONA
University of Arizona Cancer Center*
1501 North Campbell Avenue
Tucson, AZ 85724
(520) 626-6372

CALIFORNIA
USC/Norris Comprehensive Cancer
    Center*
University of Southern California
1441 Eastlake Avenue
Los Angeles, CA 90033-0804
(213) 226-2370

Jonsson Comprehensive Cancer
    Center
University of California at Los Angeles
100 UCLA Medical Plaza, Suite 255
Los Angeles, CA 90024-1781
1-800-825-2631

City Of Hope National Medical
    Center**
Beckman Research Institute
1500 East Duarte Road
Duarte, CA 91010
(818) 359-8111

University of California at San Diego
    Cancer Center**
225 Dickinson Street
San Diego, CA 92103
(619) 543-6178

COLORADO
University of Colorado Cancer
   Center**
4200 East Ninth Avenue, Box B188
Denver, CO 80262
(303) 270-3007

CONNECTICUT
Yale University Comprehensive
   Cancer Center*
333 Cedar Street
New Haven, CT 06510
(203) 785-4095

DISTRICT OF COLUMBIA
Lombardi Cancer Research Center*
Georgetown University Medical
   Center
3800 Reservoir Road, N.W.
Washington, DC 20007
(202) 687-2192

FLORIDA
Sylvester Comprehensive Cancer
   Center*
University of Miami Medical School
1475 Northwest 12th Avenue
Miami, FL 33136
(305) 545-1000

ILLINOIS
Robert H. Lurie Cancer Center**
Northwestern University
303 East Chicago Avenue
Olson Pavilion, Room 8250
Chicago, IL 60611
(312) 908-8400

University of Chicago Cancer Research
   Center**
5841 South Maryland Avenue
Chicago, IL 60637
(312) 702-9200

MARYLAND
The Johns Hopkins Oncology Center*
600 North Wolfe Street, Room B156
Baltimore, MD 21287-8915
(410) 955-8964

MASSACHUSETTS
Dana Farber Cancer Institute*
44 Binney Street
Boston, MA 02115
(617) 632-3476

MICHIGAN
Meyer L. Prentis Comprehensive
   Cancer Center of Metropolitan
   Detroit*
110 East Warren Avenue
Detroit, MI 48201
(313) 745-4329

University of Michigan
   Comprehensive Cancer Center*
101 Simpson Drive
Ann Arbor, MI 48109-0752
(313) 936-9583

MINNESOTA
Mayo Comprehensive Cancer Center*
200 First Street Southwest
Rochester, MN 55902
(507) 284-3413

NEW HAMPSHIRE
Norris Cotton Cancer Center*
Dartmouth Hitchcock Medical Center
2 Maynard Street
Hanover, NH 03756
(603) 646-5505

NEW YORK
Memorial Sloan-Kettering Cancer
    Center*
1275 York Avenue
New York, NY 10021
1-800-525-2225

Roswell Park Cancer Institute*
Elm and Carlton Streets
Buffalo, NY 14263
1-800-ROSWELL (1-800-767-9355)

Kaplan Cancer Center*
New York University Medical Center
462 First Avenue
New York, NY 10016-9103
(212) 263-6485

Columbia University Cancer Center**
College of Physicians and Surgeons
630 West 168th Street
New York, NY 10032
(212) 305-6905

Albert Einstein College of Medicine**
Cancer Research Center
Chanin Building
1300 Morris Park Avenue
Bronx, NY 10461
(718) 920-4826

University of Rochester Cancer
    Center**
601 Elmwood Avenue, Box 704
Rochester, NY 14642
(716) 275-4911

NORTH CAROLINA
Duke Comprehensive Cancer Center*
Post Office Box 3814
Durham, NC 27710
(919) 684-2748

UNC Lineberger Comprehensive
    Cancer Center*
University of North Carolina School
    of Medicine
Chapel Hill, NC 27599
(919) 966-4431

Cancer Center of Wake Forest
    University
Bowman Gray School of Medicine*
300 South Hawthorne Road
Winston Salem, NC 27103
(919) 748-4354

OHIO
Ohio State University Comprehensive
    Cancer Center*
Arthur G. James Cancer Hospital
410 West 10th Avenue
Columbus, OH 43210
1-800-638-6996

Ireland Cancer Center at Case
    Western Reserve University**
University Hospitals of Cleveland
2074 Abington Road
Cleveland, OH 44106
(216) 844-5432

PENNSYLVANIA
Fox Chase Cancer Center*
7701 Burholme Avenue
Philadelphia, PA 19111
(215) 728-2570

University of Pennsylvania Cancer
    Center*
3400 Civic Center Blvd.
6 Penn Tower
Philadelphia, PA 19104
(215) 662-3914

Pittsburgh Cancer Institute*
200 Meyran Avenue
Pittsburgh, PA 15213-2592
1-800-537-4063

TENNESSEE
St. Jude Children's Research
    Hospital**
332 North Lauderdale Street
Memphis, TN 38101-0318
(901) 522-0306

Drew Meharry Morehouse
    Consortium Cancer Center
1005 D.B. Todd Boulevard
Nashville, TN 37208
(615) 327-6927

TEXAS
The University of Texas
    M.D. Anderson Cancer Center*
1515 Holcombe Boulevard
Houston, TX 77030
(713) 792-3245

San Antonio Cancer Institute**
4450 Medical Drive
San Antonio, TX 78229
(210) 616-5798

UTAH
Utah Cancer Center**
University of Utah School of Medicine
50 North Medical Drive,
    Room 2C 110
Salt Lake City, UT 84132
(801)-581-4048

VERMONT
Vermont Regional Cancer Center*
University of Vermont
1 South Prospect Street
Burlington, VT 05401
(802) 656-4580

VIRGINIA
Massey Cancer Center**
Medical College of Virginia
Virginia Commonwealth University
1200 East Broad Street
Richmond, VA 23298
(804) 371-5116

WASHINGTON
Fred Hutchinson Cancer Research
    Center*
1124 Columbia Street
Seattle, WA 98104
(206) 667-5000
(Bone marrow transplantation
    primary treatment offered.)

WISCONSIN
University of Wisconsin
    Comprehensive Cancer Center*
600 Highland Avenue
Madison, WI 53792
(608) 263-8090

Basic Science Cancer Centers
Supported by the National Cancer Institute

La Jolla Cancer Research Foundation
La Jolla, California

Armand Hammer Center for Cancer Biology, Salk Institute
San Diego, California

Purdue Cancer Center, Purdue University
West Lafayette. Indiana

The Jackson Laboratory
Bar Harbor, Maine

Center for Cancer Research, Massachusetts Institute of Technology
Cambridge, Massachusetts

Eppley Institute, University of Nebraska Medical Center
Omaha, Nebraska

Cold Spring Harbor Laboratory
Cold Spring Harbor, New York

American Health Foundation
New York, New York

Wistar Institute
Philadelphia, Pennsylvania

Fels Research Institute, Temple University School of Medicine
Philadelphia, Pennsylvania

Cancer Center, University of Virginia Health Sciences Center
Charlottesville, Virginia

McArdle Laboratory for Cancer Research, University of Wisconsin
Madison, Wisconsin

Appendix G

NCI Clinical Trials Cooperative Group Program

The Clinical Trials Cooperative Group Program (CTCGP) is sponsored by the National Cancer Institute (NCI). It is designed to promote and support clinical trials of new cancer treatments, to explore methods of cancer prevention and early detection, and to study quality of life issues and rehabilitation during and after treatment.

Cooperative groups are composed of academic institutions and cancer treatment centers throughout the United States, Canada and Europe. They work with NCI to identify important questions in cancer research and to design carefully controlled clinical trials to answer these questions.

"The cooperative groups have been instrumental in developing new standards of cancer patient management and sophisticated clinical trials techniques," says the director of the Clinical Trials Cooperative Group Program, Richard S. Ungerleider, M.D. "They have brought us answers to numerous questions about the treatment of cancer."

There are 14 major cooperative groups, involving more than 2,200 institutions that contribute patients to group conducted clinical trials. More than 16,000 individual investigators also participate in NCI-supported cooperative group studies.

The groups differ in structure and research focus. Some groups, such as the Brain Tumor Cooperative Group, concentrate on treatment of a single type of cancer. Some, such as the Radiation Therapy Oncology Group, study a specific type of cancer therapy. Others, such as the Gynecologic Oncology Group, focus on a group of related cancers. The groups share a common purpose—to develop and conduct large scale trials in multi-institutional settings.

A patient who is interested in taking part in a trial should talk with his or her doctor. Doctors can obtain up-to-date information from PDQ, NCI's database of cancer information. Patients can call Cancer Information Service, 1-800-4-CANCER (1-800-422-6237). Staff at the CIS can answer questions in English or Spanish and will send free printed material about cancer. In addition, CIS offices serve specific geographic areas and have information about cancer-related services and resources in their region.

Clinical Trials Cooperative Groups

Brain Tumor Cooperative Group
William R. Shapiro, M.D., Chair
Barrow Neurological Institute
St. Joseph Hospital and Medical
   Center
350 West Thomas Road
Phoenix, AZ 85013

Cancer and Leukemia Group B
O. Ross McIntyre, M.D., Chair
Central Office of the Chair
Suite 2
444 Mount Support Road
Rural Route 3, Box 750
Lebanon, NH 03766

Children's Cancer Group
W. Archie Bleyer, M.D., Chair
Department of Pediatrics, Box 87
University of Texas M.D. Anderson
   Cancer Center
1515 Holcombe Boulevard
Houston, TX 77030

Eastern Cooperative Oncology Group
Douglass Tormey, M.D., Chair
AMC Cancer Research Center
1600 Pierce Street
Denver, CO 80214

European Organization for Research
   on Treatment for Cancer
Francoise Meunier, M.D., Director
EORTC Central Office—Data Center
Avenue E. Mounier 83, BTE 11
1200 Brussels, Belgium

Gynecologic Oncology Group
Robert C. Park, M.D., Chair
GOG Central Office, Suite 1945
1234 Market Street
Philadelphia, PA 19107

Intergroup Rhabdomyosarcoma Study
Harold M. Maurer, M.D., Chair
Dean's Office
University of Nebraska College of
   Medicine
600 South 42nd Street
Omaha, NE 68198-6545

National Surgical Adjuvant Breast and
   Bowel Project
Ronald Herberman, M.D., Chair
University of Pittsburgh
914 Scaife Hall
3550 Terrace Street
Pittsburgh, PA 15261

National Wilms' Tumor Study Group
Daniel M. Green, M.D., Chair
Roswell Park Cancer Institute
Elm and Carlton Streets
Buffalo, NY 14263

North Central Cancer Treatment
   Group
Michael J. O'Connell, M.D., Chair
Mayo Foundation
200 First Street, SW
Rochester, MN 55905

Pediatric Oncology Group
Sharon B. Murphy, M.D., Chair
Suite 910
645 North Michigan Avenue
Chicago, IL 60611

Quality Assurance Review Center
Arvin S. Glicksman, M.D., Chair
Quality Assurance Review Center
Roger Williams General Hospital
825 Chalkstone Avenue
Providence, RI 02908

Radiation Therapy Oncology Group
James Cox, M.D., Chair
University of Texas M.D. Anderson
   Cancer Center
1515 Holcombe Boulevard
Houston, TX 77030

Southwest Oncology Group
Charles A. Coltman, M.D., Chair
14980 Omicron Drive
San Antonio, TX 78245-3217

NOTES

(Only the first author of each work is provided. NCI is the National Cancer Institute. ACS is the American Cancer Society. JAMA is the Journal of the American Medical Association. The last number in each entry is the page number.)

Chapter 1. The Digestive Puzzle

1. R. McAllister, *Cancer* (New York: Basic Books, 1993), 156.
2. NCI, *What You Need to Know About Cancer of the Colon and Rectum* (Publication #90-1552, 1989), 2.
3. NCI, *Colon Cancer* (PDQ, Aug 1993), 1.
4. NCI, *Cancer of the Colon and Rectum* (Publication #92-95, Oct 1991), 2.
5. American Cancer Society, *Colostomy—A Guide* (Publication #4703, 1991), 6.
6. J. DeCosse, *Cancer Book* (New York: Doubleday, 1986), 342-343.
7. ACS, *Facts on Colorectal Cancer* (Publication #2004-LE, 1993), 1.
8. NCI, *Cancer of the Colon and Rectum* (Publication #92-95, Oct 1991), 2.

Chapter 2. Polyps & Bowel Cancer

1. J. Johnson, *Staying Healthy With Cancer* (Minnetonka, MN: Chronimed Publishing, 1994), 9.
2. NCI, *Cancer of the Colon and Rectum* (Publication #92-95, Oct 1991), 3.
3. ACS, *Cancer Facts and Figures—1994*, 1.
4. NCI, *What You Need to Know About Cancer of the Colon and Rectum* (Publication #90-1552, 1989), 3.
5. M. Dollinger, *Everyone's Guide to Cancer Therapy* (Toronto: Andrews & McMeed, 1991), 312-315.
6. "Bowel Cancer: Nipping it in the Bud," *Harvard Medical School Health Letter* (Sep 1989), 1.
7. D. Fleischer, "Detection and Surveillance of Colorectal Cancer," *JAMA* (Jan 27, 1989), 580-585.
8. NCI, *Cancer of the Colon and Rectum* (Publication #92-95, Oct 1991), 8.
9. K. Knight, "Occult Blood Screening for Colorectal Cancer," *JAMA* (Jan 27, 1989), 586-589.
10. "Positive for Occult Blood: What Next?" *Patient Care* (Dec 15, 1991), 167-168.
11. "Bowel Cancer: Nipping it in the Bud," *Harvard Medical School Health Letter* (Sep 1989), 1.
12. M. Dollinger, *Everyone's Guide to Cancer Therapy* (Toronto: Andrews & McMeed, 1991), 312-315.
13. "Bowel Cancer: Nipping it in the Bud," *Harvard Medical School Health Letter* (Sep 1989), 1.
14. J. Hardcastle, Colorectal Cancer: *Textbook for General Practitioners* (New York: Springer-Verlag, 1993), 22.
15. D. Lieberman, "Screening/Early Detection Model for Colorectal Cancer," *Cancer Supplement* (Oct 1, 1994), 2023-2026.

16. "Bowel Cancer: Nipping it in the Bud," *Harvard Medical School Health Letter* (Sep 1989), 1.
17. ACS, *Facts on Colorectal Cancer* (Publication #2004-LE, 1993), 3.
18. NCI, *Cancer of the Colon and Rectum* (Publication #92-95, Oct 1991), 1.
19. ACS, *Facts on Colorectal Cancer* (Publication #2004-LE, 1993), 1.
20. ACS, *Cancer Facts and Figures*—1995, 6.
21. ACS, *Facts on Colorectal Cancer* (Publication #2004-LE, 1993), 3.
22. J. Selby, "Sigmoidoscopy in the Periodic Health Examination of Asymptomatic Adults," *JAMA* (Jan 27, 1989), 595-601.
23. D. Fleischer, "Detection and Surveillance of Colorectal Cancer," *JAMA* (Jan. 27, 1989), 580-585.
24. J. Hardcastle, *Colorectal Cancer: Textbook for General Practitioners* (New York: Springer-Verlag, 1993), 22.
25. J. DeCosse, "Colorectal Cancer: Detection, Treatment, and Rehabilitation," *A Cancer Journal for Clinicians* (Jan/Feb 1994), 27-37.
26. J. DeCosse, "Colorectal Cancer: Detection, Treatment, and Rehabilitation," *A Cancer Journal for Clinicians* (Jan/Feb 1994), 27-37.
27. D. Eddy, "Screening Cancer in a High Risk Population," *Gastroenterology* (Nov 1987), 682-687.
28. D. Fleischer, "Detection and Surveillance of Colorectal Cancer," *JAMA* (Jan 27, 1989), 580-585.
29. J. DeCosse, "Colorectal Cancer: Detection, Treatment, and Rehabilitation," *A Cancer Journal for Clinicians* (Jan/Feb 1994), 27-37.
30. ACS, *Cancer Facts and Figures*—1994, 13.
31. ACS, *Cancer Facts and Figures*—1994, 11.
32. ACS, *Cancer Facts and Figures*—1995, 6.
33. NCI, *Diet and Large-Bowel Cancer—The Facts Behind the PPT* (1994), 2.
34. "Bowel Cancer: Nipping it in the Bud," *Harvard Medical School Health Letter* (Sep 1989), 1.
35. ACS, *Cancer Facts and Figures*—1995, 6.
36. K. Smigel, "Group Defines Directions for Colorectal Cancer Screening," *Journal of the National Cancer Institute* (July 6, 1994), 958-960.
37. J. DeCosse, "Colorectal Cancer: Detection, Treatment, and Rehabilitation," *A Cancer Journal for Clinicians* (Jan/Feb 1994), 27-37.

Chapter 3. Polyp Form & the Spread of Cancer

1. *Stedman's Medical Dictionary* (Baltimore: William Wood and Company, 1990), 899-902.
2. NCI, *What You Need to Know About Cancer of the Colon and Rectum* (Publication #90-1552, 1989), 6.
3. *Webster's Medical Desk Dictionary* (Springfield, MA: Merriam-Webster Inc., 1986), 430.
4. NCI, *Cancer of the Colon and Rectum* (Publication #92-95, Oct 1991), 17.
5. P. Turk, "Results of Surgical Treatment of Nonhepatic Recurrence of Colorectal Cancer," *Cancer Supplement* (Jan 15, 1993), 426-427.

6. NCI, *What You Need to Know About Cancer of the Colon and Rectum* (Publication #90-1552, 1989), 17.

7. ACS, *The Cancer Book* (New York: Doubleday, 1986), 625.

8. T. Allen-Mersh, "Colorectal Cancer—Diagnosis, Management and Prognosis," *Comprehensive Therapy* (Jan 1991), 3-7.

9. M. Dollinger, *Everyone's Guide to Cancer Therapy* (Toronto: Andrews & McMeed, 1991), 312-325.

10. NCI, *Cancer of the Colon and Rectum* (Publication #92-95, Oct 1991), 17.

11. NCI, *Cancer of the Colon and Rectum* (Publication #92-95, Oct 1991), 17.

12. M. Dollinger, *Everyone's Guide to Cancer Therapy* (Toronto: Andrews & McMeed, 1991), 312-325.

13. ACS, *Colorectal Cancer: Staging* (Publication #409568, Sep 1993).

14. "Bowel Cancer: Nipping it in the Bud," *Harvard Medical School Health Letter* (Sep 1989), 1.

15. "Positive for Occult Blood: What Next?" *Patient Care* (Dec 15, 1991), 167-168.

16. E. Ferguson, "Preventing Colorectal Cancer," *Southern Medical Journal* (Nov 1990), 1295-1298.

17. J. DeCosse, "Colorectal Cancer: Detection, Treatment, and Rehabilitation," *A Cancer Journal for Clinicians* (Jan/Feb 1994), 27-37.

18. "Bowel Cancer: Nipping it in the Bud," *Harvard Medical School Health Letter* (Sep 1989), 1.

Chapter 4. Screening Methods

1. NCI, *Colon Cancer* (PDQ, Aug 1993).

2. NCI, *Cancer of the Colon and Rectum* (Publication #92-95, Oct 1991), 14.

3. ACS, *Cancer Facts and Figures—1994*, 9.

4. ACS, *Cancer Facts and Figures—1994*, 9.

5. K. Knight, "Occult Blood Screening For Colorectal Cancer." *JAMA* (Jan 27, 1989), 586-590.

6. "Positive for Occult Blood, What Next?" *Patient Care* (Dec 15, 1991), 167-168.

7. D. Fleischer, "Detection And Surveillance Of Colorectal Cancer." *JAMA* (Jan 27, 1989), 580-585.

8. D. Fleischer, "Detection And Surveillance Of Colorectal Cancer." *JAMA* (Jan 27, 1989), 580-585.

9. J. Brody, "Report Calls Simple Test Effective in Reducing Colon Cancer Deaths," The New York Times (May 13, 1993), 1.

10. D. Fleischer, "Detection And Surveillance Of Colorectal Cancer." JAMA (Jan 27, 1989), 580-585.

11. J. Brody, "Report Calls Simple Test Effective in Reducing Colon Cancer Deaths," *The New York Times* (May 13, 1993), 1.

12. J. Brody, "Report Calls Simple Test Effective in Reducing Colon Cancer Deaths," *The New York Times* (May 13, 1993), 1.

13. D. Fleischer, "Detection And Surveillance Of Colorectal Cancer." *JAMA* (Jan 27, 1989), 580-585.

14. M. MacCarty, "Colorectal Cancer: The Case For Barium Enema." *Mayo Clinic Proceedings* (Mar 1992), 253-257.
15. K. Knight, "Occult Blood Screening For Colorectal Cancer." *JAMA* (Jan 27, 1989), 586-590.
16. NCI, *Cancer of the Colon and Rectum* (Publication #92-95, Oct 1991), 14.
17. NCI, *Cancer of the Colon and Rectum* (Publication #92-95, Oct 1991), 14.
18. NCI, *Cancer of the Colon and Rectum* (Publication #92-95, Oct 1991), 14.
19. D. Fleischer, "Detection And Surveillance Of Colorectal Cancer." *JAMA* (Jan 27, 1989), 580-585.
20. NCI, *Cancer of the Colon and Rectum* (Publication #92-95, Oct 1991), 16.
21. D. Fleischer, "Detection And Surveillance Of Colorectal Cancer." *JAMA* (Jan 27, 1989), 580-585.

Chapter 5. Symptoms That Force Action

1. ACS, *Facts on Colorectal Cancer*, (Publication #2004-LE, 1993), 4.
2. NCI, *Cancer of the Colon and Rectum* (Publication #92-95, Oct 1991), 15.
3. ACS, *Cancer Facts and Figures—1994*, 9.

Chapter 6. Diagnosis

1. ACS, *Facts on Colorectal Cancer* (Publication #2004-LE, 1993), 6.
2. American Society of Colon and Rectal Surgeons, *Your Doctor is a Colon and Rectal Surgeon* (1990), 1.
3. D. Ranschoff, "Screening for Colorectal Cancer," *The New England Journal of Medicine* (July 4, 1991), 37-41.
4. D. Whynes, "Cost Savings in Mass Population Screening for Colorectal Cancer Resulting From the Early Detection and Excision of Adenomas," *Health Economics* (Apr 1992), 53-61.
5. NCI, *Cancer of the Colon and Rectum* (Publication #92-95, Oct 1991), 16.
6. NCI, *Cancer of the Colon and Rectum* (Publication #92-95, Oct 1991), 16.
7. ACS, *Colorectal Cancer: Diagnosis* (Publication #409576, Aug 1993)
8. "Positive for Occult Blood: What Next?" *Patient Care* (Dec 15, 1991), 167-168.
9. D. Fleischer, "Detection And Surveillance Of Colorectal Cancer." *JAMA* (Jan 27, 1989), 580-585.
10. D. Fleischer, "Detection And Surveillance Of Colorectal Cancer." *JAMA* (Jan 27, 1989), 580-585.
11. "Colonoscopy in Asympotomatic Patients," *Patient Care* (Apr 30, 1991), 23-24.
12. NCI, *Cancer of the Colon and Rectum* (Publication #92-95, Oct 1991), 14.
13. NCI, "Colonoscopies and Polyp Removal Help Prevent Cancer," *To Your Health ... News from the Polyp Prevention Trial* (1994).
14. T. Allen-Mersh, "Colorectal Cancer—Diagnosis, Management and Prognosis," *Comprehensive Therapy* (Jan 1991), 3-7.
15. M. MacCarty, "Colorectal Cancer: The Case For Barium Enema," *Mayo Clinic Proceedings* (March 1992), 253-257.

16. ACS, *Colorectal Cancer: Diagnosis* (Publication #409576, Aug 1993).
17. "Test After Colon Surgery Is Ineffective, Study Says," *The New York Times* (Aug 25, 1993), B7.
18. H. Asburn, "Management of Recurrent and Metastatic Colorectal Carcinoma." *Surgical Clinics of North America* (Feb 1993), 143-165.

Chapter 7. Sigmoidoscopy versus Colonoscopy

1. ACS, *Facts on Colorectal Cancer* (Publication #2004-LE, 1993), 6.
2. "Colonoscopy in Asymptomatic Patients," *Patient Care* (Apr 30, 1991), 23-24.
3. "Positive for Occult Blood: What Next?" *Patient Care* (Dec 15, 1991), 167-168
4. "Colonoscopy in Asymptomatic Patients," *Patient Care* (Apr 30, 1991), 23-24.
5. "Positive for Occult Blood: What Next?" *Patient Care* (Dec 15, 1991), 167-168.

Chapter 8. Treatment

1. NCI, *Colon Cancer* (PDQ, Aug 1993), 5.
2. NCI, *Cancer of the Colon and Rectum* (Publication #92-95, Oct 1991), 19.
3. J. DeCosse, "Colorectal Cancer: Detection, Treatment, and Rehabilitation," *A Cancer Journal for Clinicians* (Jan/Feb 1994), 27-37.
4. ACS, *Colorectal Cancer: Treatment* (publication #409577, Aug 1993), 2.
5. NCI, *Cancer of the Colon and Rectum* (Publication #92-95, Oct 1991), 20.
6. ACS, *Colostomy—A Guide* (Publication #4703, Feb 1991), 5.
7. NCI, *What You Need to Know About Cancer of the Colon and Rectum* (Publication #90-1552, Nov 1989), 8-9.
8. ACS, *Colostomy—A Guide* (Publication #4703, Feb 1991), 44.
9. ACS, *Colostomy—A Guide* (Publication #4703, Feb 1991), 3.
10. ACS, *Colostomy—A Guide* (Publication #4703, Feb 1991), 4.
11. ACS, *Colostomy—A Guide* (Publication #4703, Feb 1991), 3.
12. NCI, *What You Need to Know About Cancer of the Colon and Rectum* (Publication #90-1552, Nov 1989), 8-9.
13. E. Ferguson, "Preventing Colorectal Cancer," *Southern Medical Journal* (Nov 1990), 1295-1298.
14. V. DeVita, Jr., *Cancer: Principles and Practice Of Oncology* (Philadelphia: J. B. Lippincott Company, 1993), 983-984.
15. NCI, *Colorectal Cancer: Treatment Overview* (Publication #409577, Oct 1993), 3.
16. NCI, *What You Need to Know About Cancer of the Colon and Rectum* (Publication #90-1552, Nov 1989), 17.
17. ACS, *Facts on Colorectal Cancer* (Publication #2004-LE, 1993), 8.
18. ACS, *Facts on Colorectal Cancer* (Publication #2004-LE, 1993), 8.
19. ACS, *Colorectal Cancer: Diagnosis* (Publication #409576, 1993), 4.

20. ACS, *Facts on Colorectal Cancer* (Publication #2004-LE, 1993), 8.
21. ACS, *Colorectal Cancer: Treatment* (Publication #409577, Aug 1993), 4.
22. NCI, *What You Need to Know About Cancer of the Colon and Rectum* (Publication #90-1552, Nov 1989), 9.
23. NCI, *What You Need to Know About Cancer of the Colon and Rectum* (Publication #90-1552, Nov 1989), 10.
24. NCI, *Cancer of the Colon and Rectum* (Publication #92-95, Oct 1991), 21-23
25. NCI, *Cancer Facts—Biological Therapies: Newest Form of Cancer Treatment* (Ref. #7.2, 1988), 3.
26. NCI, *Cancer of the Colon and Rectum* (Publication #92-95, Oct. 1991), 23.
27. NCI, *What You Need to Know About Cancer of the Colon and Rectum* (Publication #90-1552, Nov 1989), 17.
28. NCI, *What You Need to Know About Cancer of the Colon and Rectum* (Publication #90-1552, Nov 1989), 9.
29. E. Ferguson, "Preventing Colorectal Cancer," *Southern Medical Journal* (Nov 1990), 1295-1298.
30. NCI, *Cancer of the Colon and Rectum* (Publication #92-95, Oct 1991), 20.
31. J. DeCosse, "Colorectal Cancer: Detection, Treatment, and Rehabilitation," *A Cancer Journal for Clinicians* (Jan/Feb 1994), 27-37.
32. ACS, *Colorectal Cancer: Treatment* (Publication #409577, Aug 1993).
33. A. Vernova, "Current Follow-Up Strategies After Resection of Colon Cancer," *Diseases of the Colon and Rectum* (June 1994), 578-583.
34. A. Vernova, "Current Follow-Up Strategies After Resection of Colon Cancer," *Diseases of the Colon and Rectum* (June 1994), 578-583.
35. H. Asburn, "Management of Recurrent and Metastatic Colorectal Carcinoma." *Surgical Clinics of North America* (Feb. 1993), 145-165.
36. NCI, *Cancer of the Colon and Rectum* (Publication #92-95, Oct 1991), 17.
37. J. DeCosse, "Colorectal Cancer: Detection, Treatment, and Rehabilitation," *A Cancer Journal for Clinicians* (Jan/Feb 1994), 27-37.
38. A. Vernova, "Current Follow-Up Strategies After Resection of Colon Cancer," *Diseases of the Colon and Rectum* (June 1994), 578-583.
39. J. DeCosse, "Colorectal Cancer: Detection, Treatment, and Rehabilitation," *A Cancer Journal for Clinicians* (Jan/Feb 1994), 27-37.
40. ACS, *Adjuvant Treatment* (Publication #5011, 1993).
41. NCI, *What Are Clinical Trials All About?* (Publication #92-2706, June 1992)
42. NCI, *Cancer of the Colon and Rectum* (Publication #92-95, Oct 1991), 27.

Chapter 9. Prognosis

1. "Bowel Cancer: Nipping It In the Bud," *Harvard Medical School Health Letter* (Sep 1989).
2. J. Hardcastle, *Colorectal Cancer: Textbook for General Practitioners* (New York: Springer-Verlag, 1993), 17.
3. NCI, *Cancer of the Colon and Rectum* (Publication #92-95, Oct 1991), 12.
4. NCI, *Colon Cancer Prognosis* (PDQ, Aug 1994).

5. "Bowel Cancer: Nipping It In the Bud." *Harvard Medical School Health Letter* (Sep 1989).
6. NCI, *Cancer of the Colon and Rectum* (Publication #92-95, Oct 1991), 17-26.
7. M. Dollinger, *Everyone's Guide to Cancer Therapy* (Toronto: Andrews & McMeed, 1991), 312-325.
8. ACS, *Colorectal Cancer: Staging* (Publication #409568, Sep 1993).
9. J. DeCosse, "Colorectal Cancer: Detection, Treatment, and Rehabilitation," *A Cancer Journal for Clinicians* (Jan/Feb 1994), 27-37.
10. A. Vernova, "Current Follow-Up Strategies After Resection of Colon Cancer," *Diseases of the Colon and Rectum* (June 1994), 578-583.
11. NCI, *Diagnosis, Colon Cancer* (PDQ, Aug 1994).
12. NCI, *Diagnosis, Rectal Cancer* (PDQ, Dec 1994).
13. NCI, *Diagnosis, Colon Cancer* (PDQ, Aug 1994).
14. NCI, *Diagnosis, Rectal Cancer* (PDQ, Dec 1994).
15. NCI, *Cancer of the Colon and Rectum* (Publication #92-95, Oct 1991), 19-26.
16. J. DeCosse, "Colorectal Cancer: Detection, Treatment, and Rehabilitation," *A Cancer Journal for Clinicians* (Jan/Feb 1994), 27-37.
17. NCI, *Diagnosis, Colon Cancer* (PDQ, Aug 1994).
18. NCI, *Diagnosis, Rectal Cancer* (PDQ, Dec 1994).
19. NCI, *Diagnosis, Colon Cancer* (PDQ, Aug 1994).
20. NCI, *Cancer of the Colon and Rectum* (Publication #92-95, Oct 1991), 24.
21. V. DeVita, Jr., *Cancer: Principles And Practice Of Oncology* (Philadelphia: J.B. Lippincott Company, 1993), 984.
22. NCI, *Diagnosis, Colon Cancer* (PDQ, Aug 1994).
23. NCI, *Diagnosis, Rectal Cancer* (PDQ, Dec 1994).
24. NCI, *Diagnosis, Colon Cancer* (PDQ, Aug 1994).
25. NCI, *Diagnosis, Rectal Cancer* (PDQ, Dec 1994).
26. M. Dollinger, *Everyone's Guide to Cancer Therapy* (Toronto: Andrews & McMeed, 1991), 312-325.
27. J. De Cosse, "Colorectal Cancer: Detection, Treatment, and Rehabilitation." *A Cancer Journal For Clinicians* (Jan/Feb 1994), 27-37.
28. NCI, *Diagnosis, Colon Cancer* (PDQ, Aug 1994).
29. NCI, *Diagnosis, Rectal Cancer* (PDQ, Dec 1994).
30. NCI, *Diagnosis, Colon Cancer* (PDQ, Aug 1994).
31. NCI, *Diagnosis, Rectal Cancer* (PDQ, Dec 1994).
32. NCI, *Diagnosis, Colon Cancer* (PDQ, Aug 1994).
33. NCI, *Cancer of the Colon and Rectum* (Publication #92-95, Oct 1991), 21.
34. J. DeCosse, "Colorectal Cancer: Detection, Treatment, and Rehabilitation," *A Cancer Journal for Clinicians* (Jan/Feb 1994), 27-37.
35. NCI, *Diagnosis, Rectal Cancer* (PDQ, Dec 1994).
36. NCI, *Diagnosis, Colon Cancer* (PDQ, Aug 1994).
37. NCI, *Diagnosis, Rectal Cancer* (PDQ, Dec 1994).
38. NCI, *Diagnosis, Colon Cancer* (PDQ, Aug 1994).
39. NCI, *Diagnosis, Rectal Cancer* (PDQ, Dec 1994).

40. W. Forman, "The Role of Chemotherapy and Adjuvant Therapy in the Management of Colorectal Cancer," *Cancer Supplement* (Oct 1, 1994), 2151-2153.
41. W. Forman, "The Role of Chemotherapy and Adjuvant Therapy in the Management of Colorectal Cancer," *Cancer Supplement* (Oct 1, 1994), 2151-2153.
42. H. Asburn, "Management of Recurrent and Metastatic Colorectal Cancer," *Surgical Clinics of North America* (Feb 1993), 145.
43. J. DeCosse, "Colorectal Cancer: Detection, Treatment, and Rehabilitation," *A Cancer Journal for Clinicians* (Jan/Feb 1994), 27-37.
44. J. DeCosse, "Colorectal Cancer: Detection, Treatment, and Rehabilitation," *A Cancer Journal for Clinicians* (Jan/Feb 1994), 27-37.
45. H. Asburn, "Management of Recurrent and Metastatic Colorectal Cancer," *Surgical Clinics of North America* (Feb 1993), 143-165.
46. H. Asburn, "Management of Recurrent and Metastatic Colorectal Cancer," *Surgical Clinics of North America* (Feb 1993), 143-165.
47. H. Asburn, "Management of Recurrent and Metastatic Colorectal Cancer," *Surgical Clinics of North America* (Feb 1993), 143-165.
48. M. Dollinger, *Everyone's Guide to Cancer Therapy* (Toronto: Andrews & McMeed, 1991), 312-315.
49. E. Ferguson, "Preventing Colorectal Cancer," *Southern Medical Journal* (Nov 1990), 1295-1298.
50. H. Asburn, "Management of Recurrent and Metastatic Colorectal Cancer," *Surgical Clinics of North America* (Feb 1993), 143-165.
51. A. Vernova, "Current Follow-Up Strategies After Resection of Colon Cancer," *Diseases of the Colon and Rectum* (June 1994), 578-583.
52. H. Asburn, "Management of Recurrent and Metastatic Colorectal Cancer," *Surgical Clinics of North America* (Feb 1993), 143-165.
53. H. Asburn, "Management of Recurrent and Metastatic Colorectal Cancer," *Surgical Clinics of North America* (Feb 1993), 143-165.
54. A. Vernova, "Current Follow-Up Strategies After Resection of Colon Cancer," *Diseases of the Colon and Rectum* (June 1994), 578-583.
55. H. Asburn, "Management of Recurrent and Metastatic Colorectal Cancer," *Surgical Clinics of North America* (Feb 1993), 143-165.
56. H. Asburn, "Management of Recurrent and Metastatic Colorectal Cancer," *Surgical Clinics of North America* (Feb 1993), 143-165.
57. M. Dollinger, *Everyone's Guide to Cancer Therapy* (Toronto: Andrews & McMeed, 1991), 312-325.
58. K. Smigel, "Group Defines Directions For Colorectal Cancer Screening," *Journal of the National Cancer Institute* (July 6, 1994), 958-960.

Glossary

Words in *italics* are defined elsewhere in this glossary.

A

Adenoma (Adenomatous Polyp)—Type of *polyp*. Develops as an abnormal growth on the surface lining and extends into the interior space of the *large bowel*. The vast majority of adenomas are *benign*. But there is a danger that they can become *malignant*. It is a widely accepted theory that the majority of *colorectal cancer* develops from adenomas. See also *Hyperplastic Polyp; Pedunculated Polyp; Sessile Polyp.*

Adenocarcinoma—Medical term for a *malignant tumor* that rises from the layer of *tissue* lining the inside of the body's organs.

Adenoma-Carcinoma Sequence—The evolving of a *benign polyp* into *cancer.*

Adenomatous Polyp—See *Adenoma.*

Adjuvant Therapy—*Treatment* used to improve the results of a patient's primary treatment. For example, if the primary treatment is surgery, *radiation, chemotherapy* or *biological therapy* can be used as adjuvant therapy. Adjuvant therapy can be utilized before, during and/or after primary treatment to destroy *cancer cells* that cannot be surgically removed. Also used to lower the risk that hidden, undetectable cancer cells may exist.

Air-Contrast Barium Enema—See *Barium Enema.*

Alternative Cancer Treatments—Nontraditional or non-medical *treatments* for *cancer.* Usually not accepted by the medical community.

Anal Canal (Anal Region)—1- to 2-inch passageway linking the *rectum* to the *anus.*

Anastomosis—In *colorectal-cancer treatment*, reconnecting the two sections of the *large bowel* after the segment containing *cancer* has been surgically removed. See also *Bowel Resection.*

Anemia—A reduction in the number of red blood cells in the body; may be a symptom of a digestive-tract problem.

Anesthesia—Loss of feeling, and thus of pain, in part of the body during surgery or other treatment.

Anorexia—Loss of appetite for food.

Antioxidants—Chemical compounds, including vitamins E and C and beta carotene, that the body uses to neutralize free radicals. Free radicals are formed during the oxidation process and have been linked to the development of cancer.

Anus—Final element in the digestive system. The external opening through which waste is passed out of the body.

Appliance—Bag used to collect waste which is eliminated through a *stoma*, a surgically created opening in the abdomen. See also *Colostomy.*

Ascorbic Acid—Vitamin C

Average Risk—Anyone who is not at *high risk* for *colorectal cancer* is considered of average risk. Depending on the medical authority, 55% to 85% of all colorectal cancer is found in people who fall into the average-risk category. Average-risk considerations begin at age 40—generally less than 3% of *polyps* and colorectal cancer are found in people under age 40. Age 50 is the turning point. Each passing decade doubles the chances that an average-risk person will be diagnosed with *adenomas* or colorectal cancer. More than 93% of people diagnosed with colorectal cancer are over 50 years of age. See also *High Risk*.

B

Barium Enema (Lower GI Series)—Diagnostic procedure that is an X-ray study of the *large bowel*. Patient is given an enema of a thick, liquid-barium mixture before X-rays are taken. On the X-ray, the barium shows a silhouette of the bowel with an outline of any *tumors* that are present. To expand the bowel and make tumors more visible, air may be pumped into the bowel during the test. This technique is called an "air-contrast" or "double-contrast barium enema" and is the procedure commonly used today because of its greater dependability.

The double-contrast barium enema is generally considered a less accurate diagnostic procedure for colorectal cancer than a *colonoscopy*. A double-contrast barium enema is sometimes used after a colonoscopy to provide an additional diagnostic perspective. When a colonoscopy is not possible, a double-contrast barium enema may be used in combination with a *sigmoidoscopy*.

Benign—Description of a tumor that shows no tendency to expand into surrounding *tissues* or spread to other parts of the body. Benign is the opposite of *malignant*. Although benign growths can interfere with normal bodily functions, they are not cancerous and generally are not considered dangerous.

Biological Therapy (Immunotherapy)—*Treatment* that uses the body's natural defense system to fight disease. Scientists have identified a number of substances called "biological-response modifiers" (BRMs) that may improve the body's normal defenses against *cancer*. Biological therapy attempts to strengthen the patient's *immune system* to fight the disease. One of the newest cancer treatments, it is now in its experimental and developmental phase.

Biopsy—Surgical removal of *tissue* from the body for laboratory analysis to determine whether or not it is cancerous. In almost all cases, a biopsy is the method used to determine whether a growth is *malignant* or *benign*.

Bowel—Part of the *digestive system*. See also *Large Bowel; Small Bowel*.

Bowel Resection—Surgery that removes the cancerous section and surrounding areas of the *bowel*, creating two separate bowel segments. After removal of the affected parts, the bowel is reattached or spliced together. The most common and preferred treatment for *colorectal cancer*, bowel resection enables the patient to resume normal body functions after the cancer is removed. Illustration on page 46. See also *Anastomosis*.

BRMs—See *Biological Therapy*.

C

Calcium—A *mineral* found in bones. A low calcium intake is one of the dietary factors associated with osteoporosis, a disease characterized by a decrease in the amount of bone, which leads to easy fractures. Primary sources are dairy products, such as milk, yogurt, cheese and ice cream, and dark-green vegetables.

Calorie—Calories measure the energy your body gets from food. The body needs calories as "fuel" to perform all of its functions, such as breathing, circulating the blood, and physical activity. When you are sick, your body may need extra calories to fight fever or other problems. Calories are derived from the *protein, fats* and *carbohydrates* in food and from alcohol. Everybody needs calories for daily living, but the amount varies for each person, depending on age, sex, height, weight and physical activity.

Cancer—General term for over 100 diseases characterized by abnormal and uncontrolled growth of *cells*. Cancer will invade normal *tissues* in the vicinity of the original *tumor*. Cancer cells can also spread via the bloodstream and *lymphatic system* to take root in healthy tissues throughout the body. See also *Metastasis*.

Carbohydrate—One of the three *nutrients* that supply *calories* (energy) to the body. Carbohydrates are needed for normal body function. There are two kinds of carbohydrates—simple (sugars) and complex (starches and fiber). Primary sources for simple carbohydrates are sugars, syrups, honey, candy, regular soft drinks, cakes and cookies. Primary sources for complex carbohydrates are whole grains (wheat, rye, oats, corn and barley), whole-grain breads and cereals, fruits, vegetables, beans and peas.

Carbohydrates are the major sources of energy for the body's internal functioning and for physical activity. They also help maintain body temperature. 55% to 60% of your total calories should come from carbohydrates, primarily complex sources. See also *Fat; Protein.*

Carcinoma—*Cancer* that develops in the *tissues* that form the lining or inner surface of organs such as the *large bowel*. From 80% to 90% of all *malignant tumors* are carcinomas. The term "carcinoma" is frequently used synonymously with "cancer."

Carcinoma in situ—Earliest stage of *cancer*. The *tumor* is confined to the area where it started, and has not yet spread or grown to a significant size. Carcinoma in situ is highly curable.

Cauterization—Destruction or cutting of tissue with an electric current; used to remove polyps during a polypectomy.

CEA Assay (Carcinoembryonic Antigen Test)—Blood test that measures substances that may be elevated and show up in the blood of a person with *colorectal cancer*. Although questions exist as to its reliability, it is widely used after colorectal-cancer surgery for detection of *recurrence*. It is not considered a useful test for *screening* purposes and may have limited value in the *diagnosis* of colorectal cancer.

Cecum—First section of the *large bowel*.

Cells—Individual living units of which all *tissues* are composed. Cells are the fundamental building blocks of human tissue, the smallest bodies capable of independent reproduction. In the normal life process, cells constantly and routinely reproduce themselves. See also *Cancer.*

Chemotherapy—*Treatment* of *cancer* by using drugs designed to destroy cancer *cells* or to stop them from growing and spreading. Drugs are given to patients by mouth or by injection into a muscle, an artery or a vein. The drugs travel through the bloodstream to almost every area of the body. See also *5-Fluorourocil.*

Clinical Trials—Organized and systematic evaluations of potential new *cancer treatments* conducted with patients.

Colon—Part of the *large bowel* between the *cecum* and the *rectum.* Divided into the ascending, transverse, descending and sigmoid sections, the colon looks like an inverted U. It begins on the right side of the body and extends up, over and down the left side. The main functions of the colon are to absorb fluids and to process and solidify the 5% to 10% of food waste that remains after food passes through the *small bowel.* Illustration on page 9. See also *Digestive System; Large Bowel.*

Colonoscopy—Examination of the *colon* with a *fiberoptic* instrument called a colonoscope. The thin, flexible, periscope-like colonoscope is inserted through the *anus,* into the *rectum,* and through the entire colon. It makes it possible for the doctor to investigate the full length of the *large bowel* visually. During the course of the colonoscopy the doctor can perform a *biopsy* or a *polypectomy.*

Colorectal Cancer—Any *cancer* that develops in the *rectum* or *colon.*

Colostomy—Surgical procedure in which an artificial opening, a *stoma,* is created in the abdomen. This allows for by-passing the excretion function of the *large bowel.* Body waste drains through the stoma into a bag. The bag, or *appliance,* is undetectable to the outside world. A colostomy is sometimes necessary after the removal of a diseased section of the colon, when *bowel resection* cannot be performed. Also utilized in cases of advanced rectal cancer or when a *tumor* develops close to the *anus,* a colostomy can be temporary or permanent. After the natural healing process, a temporary colostomy can be reversed and the patient is able to resume normal bodily functions. Fewer than 15% of all *colorectal-cancer* patients require a permanent colostomy.

D

Dehydration—An abnormal loss of water from the body. Can be caused by severe diarrhea or vomiting.

Diagnosis—The process of identifying an illness. A description of a disease or disorder. A diagnosis of *cancer* is usually followed by *staging* to determine the extent of the cancer. As a general rule, cancer can be definitively diagnosed only after a *biopsy.*

Diet—The foods a person eats, including both liquids and solids.

Dietary Fat—See *Fat.*

Digestive System (Intestinal Tract, Gastrointestinal Tract)—The parts of the body that work together to convert and process food so *nutrients* can enter the bloodstream for distribution throughout the body. The digestive system also processes, stores and disposes of waste. In the digestive system, food enters the mouth, travels down the esophagus into the stomach, through the *small bowel*, into the *large bowel*, through the *anal canal* and out the *anus*. Illustration on page 8. See also *Colon; Cecum; Rectum.*

Digital Rectal Exam—*Screening* procedure in which a doctor inserts a lubricated, gloved finger through the patient's *anus* and into the *rectum* to feel for irregular or abnormally firm growths. The doctor will also look for traces of blood in the *feces* particles that come out on the gloved finger. The rectal exam should be part of the annual physical exam after a person reaches 40 years of age.

Distal Colon (Left Colon)—The last part of the *large bowel*, including the descending colon, sigmoid colon and rectum. Illustration on page 9. See also *Colon; Proximal Colon.*

Diuretics—Drugs that help the body get rid of water and salt.

Diverticulitis—Common, usually not serious, *digestive-system* problem with *symptoms* similar to those of *colorectal cancer*. It is an *infection* or inflammation of one or several of the small pockets or sacs situated in the wall of the *colon*. It can cause tenderness, diarrhea, pain and occasionally fever. Individuals over the age of 40 have a 1-in-3 chance of experiencing diverticulitis.

Double-Contrast Barium Enema—See *Barium Enema.*

Dukes' System—*Cancer staging* system that describes the extent cancer has spread in a patient. Although there are variations, it is most common for Dukes' A to represent the start-up stage of cancer, with Dukes' B, Dukes' C and Dukes' D describing ever-worsening conditions of the disease. See also *TNM System.*

Dyspepsia (Indigestion)—Upset stomach.

Dysphagia—Difficulty in swallowing.

Dysplasia—Abnormal development in the size, shape and organization of *cells* and *tissue*. Does not always develop into *cancer*. As it relates to the *colon*, dysplasia generally refers to the slow transformation of *benign polyps* into *malignancy*. Dysplasia ceases when the *tumor* is unmistakably determined to be cancer.

E

Edema—The buildup of excess fluid within the *tissues.*

Electrocoagulation or Electrofulguration—Early-*stage treatment* for *cancer* located in the *rectum*. Uses high-frequency electrical current to destroy the *tumor.*

Electrolytes—A general term for the *minerals* necessary to give the body the proper fluid balance.

Endocavitary Irradiation—New primary *treatment* for rectal *cancer*. An X-ray tube is fitted onto an endoscopic instrument similar to those used in *colonoscopy* and *sigmoidoscopy*. Looking through the scope that has been inserted through the *anus*, the doctor can aim rays directly at the *tumor*. See also *Radiation Therapy*.

Endoscopy—General term referring to the examination of the interior of the body. *Colonoscopy* and *sigmoidoscopy* are types of endoscopic examinations. The introduction of *fiber optics* in the 1970s provided simple endoscopic methods for detecting *malignancies*, precancerous growths and non-*cancer*-related diseases and disorders without the risk of major exploratory surgery.

Enterostomal Therapy (ET) Nurse—Person who takes care of *colostomy* patients and teaches them about their *treatments* and care.

External Radiation—*Radiation therapy* that uses a machine located outside the body to aim high-energy rays at *cancer cells*. See also *Internal Radiation*.

F

Familial Polyposis—Hereditary condition that results in the growth of hundreds or sometimes thousands of *polyps* in the large *bowel*. Similar to Gardner's Syndrome. Persons with familial polyposis are at *high risk* of developing *colorectal cancer*. Familial polyposis and other genetic diseases account for less than 1% of all colorectal-cancer cases.

Fat—One of the three *nutrients* that supply *calories* (energy) to the body. Small amounts of fat are necessary for normal body function, such as helping the body absorb certain *vitamins*. Fats also form parts of body *cells* and hormones.

Fats supply a large amount of energy in a small amount of food, providing twice as many calories per ounce as *carbohydrates* and *proteins*. Foods high in fats are also high in calories. Approximately 20% to 30% of your total calories should come from fat. Primary sources of fat are meats, sausage, bacon, cream, cheese , butter, whole milk, oil, margarine and salad dressings. See also *Carbohydrate; Protein*.

Fecal Occult Blood Test (FOBT) (Occult Blood Test, Stool-Blood Test)—Chemical test to determine if there is blood in the stool. Performed at home by patient, who smears small *feces* samples from consecutive bowel movements onto chemically treated cards. These are sent to a laboratory for analysis. A positive stool-blood test indicates only that blood is in the stool, not what is causing the bleeding. This is a test for blood—not a test for *cancer*. Test should be part of the annual physical examination of everyone over 50 years of age.

Feces—Bodily waste formed in the *colon*, stored in the *rectum* and excreted through the *anus*.

Fiber, Dietary—Parts of food that are not digested but pass through the digestive system basically intact. Fiber enhances the formation and movement of stools through the large bowel and is believed to reduce the risk of developing colorectal cancer.

Fiber Optics—Technology used in the sigmoidoscope and colonoscope. These instruments consist of thin flexible tubes containing fibers capable of transmitting high-intensity light and images. With them a doctor can inspect the interior walls of the *large bowel* visually, eliminating the need for surgery to determine the condition inside the large bowel. He or she can also perform a *polypectomy* to remove small suspicious growths or cut out pieces of tissue for a *biopsy*. See also *Colonoscopy; Endoscopy; Polypectomy; Sigmoidoscopy.*

5-Fluorourocil (5-FU)—Drug used in *chemotherapy* treatment for *colorectal-cancer* patients. See also *Chemotherapy.*

FOBT—See *Fecal Occult Blood Test.*

Fortified—A food is fortified when extra *nutrients* are added.

G

Gastroenterologist—A physician who specializes in diseases and disorders of the *digestive system.*

Gene—The basic unit of heredity; one means by which diseases are passed from one generation to the next.

Glucose—A simple sugar occurring in some fruits and honey; the sugar found in blood.

H

Hemorrhoids—Common, usually not serious, medical problem that can cause *symptoms* similar to those of *colorectal cancer.* Hemorrhoids develop from swollen blood vessels. Internal hemorrhoids are situated in the *anal canal.* External hemorrhoids are found in the proximity of the *anus.* Hemorrhoids are usually treated with local ointments, sitz baths and suppositories.

High Risk—Status of an individual, referring to the probability of the person getting a certain disease such as *colorectal cancer.* High risk, in a particular age bracket, is measured against *average risk* in the same age bracket. High risk means that the chances of getting a disease are somewhat greater than that of the general population. High risk does not mean that someone will get the disease.

A person is in a high-risk category of getting colorectal cancer if he or she has been diagnosed with colorectal cancer or *adenomatous polyps* in the past or has blood relatives who had colorectal cancer or polyps. The number of relatives, the closeness of the relationships and the ages of the relatives are factors that influence the risk. The appearance of these conditions in a first-degree relative (parent, child or sibling) before age 55 is of particular significance. Other high-risk factors include the presence of long-term ulcerative colitis, *familial polyposis* or, in women, breast or ovarian cancer.

Hyperplastic Polyp—A small, common *polyp*, generally considered to be harmless. See also *Adenoma; Pedunculated Polyp; Sessile Polyp.*

I

Immune System—The parts of the body that work together to protect the body against disease. See also *Biological Therapy.*

Immunotherapy—See *Biological Therapy.*

Infection—When germs enter the body and produce disease, the disease is called an infection. Infections can occur in any part of the body. They cause a fever and other problems, depending on the site of the infection. When the body's natural defense system is strong, it can often fight the entering germs and prevent infection. *Cancer treatment* can weaken the natural defense system, but good *nutrition* can help make it stronger.

In Situ—See *Carcinoma In Situ.*

Internal Radiation—Type of treatment in which the source of the radiation is implanted into or near the area being treated. See also *External Radiation; Radiation Therapy.*

Internist—General classification of doctors who treat a wide range of internal medical problems. Sub-specialists listed within the broad classification of internists include *gastroenterologists* and *oncologists.*

Intravenous (IV) feeding—Giving a patient some of the *nutrients* he or she needs through a needle in a vein. IV feeding is used when a person is unable to eat solid food, such as right after surgery.

Invasive Cancer—Cancer that spreads to the healthy *tissue* surrounding the original *tumor* site.

L

Lactose Intolerance— Difficulty in digesting lactose, a sugar in milk. May occur after some types of surgery. Lactose intolerance may go away over time. There are special milk products available without lactose.

Large Bowel (Large Intestine)—Tubular organ, 1.5 to 1.8 meters (5 to 6 feet) long and 2.5 to 7.5cm (1 to 3 inches) in diameter. Comprised of the *cecum*, the *colon* and the *rectum*, it is situated at the end of the *digestive system*. The main function of the large bowel is to process food waste by solidifying, storing and excreting it. Illustration on page 9. See also *Small Bowel.*

Laser Therapy—Using an intense beam of radiation (laser) to reduce the size of a tumor.

Left Colon—See *Distal Colon.*

Lesion—Any abnormal change in the surface of an organ such as the *large bowel*. Term used synonymously with *tumor, neoplasm* and *polyp.*

Local Excision—Surgical procedure sometimes used for *cancer* in early *stages.* The surgeon uses a tube-shaped instrument inserted through the *anus* to cut out *tumors* lodged in the *rectum* or lower portion of the *colon.*

Lower GI Series—See *Barium Enema.*

Lymph Fluid, Lymph Nodes, Lymphatic System—The body's lymphatic system normally acts as the first natural defense against germs. It produces and stores *infection*-fighting cells, which circulate through the body in the lymph fluid. The lymphatic circulation system is composed of vessels similar to blood vessels, through which lymph fluid circulates.

The small, rounded, bean-shaped lymph nodes, also called lymph glands, are situated at frequent intervals throughout the lymph circulation system.

The lymph fluid is purified as it passes through the lymph nodes, which filter out and destroy waste, bacteria and foreign substances.

Cancer cells can spread throughout the body via the lymphatic system as well as the bloodstream. In the lymph system, cancer cells can be transported to the nearest lymph nodes, where they can take root and begin to grow. Because the lymph system flows into the bloodstream, there is also the possibility that cancer in the lymph nodes will spread to the body's organs via the bloodstream. In addition to removing cancerous areas during surgery, surrounding *tissues* and nearby lymph nodes are often taken out to determine whether cancer has spread from the original site.

M

Malignant—Cancerous; the opposite of *benign. Malignant tumor* and *cancer* mean the same thing. Malignant *cells* have four important characteristics—a relentless tendency to divide and reproduce; behavior that interferes with the functions of healthy cells; a strong inclination to sink roots into surrounding *tissues*; and the inherent danger of spreading elsewhere via the bloodstream or *lymphatic system.* See also *Metastasis.*

Malnutrition—The condition resulting when the body receives too few of the essential *nutrients.*

Metastasis (Secondary Cancer)—Spread of the original *cancer* from one part of the body to another. Examined under a microscope, the cancer *cells* that form the secondary *tumors* are like the cells of the primary or original tumor. For *colorectal cancer,* metastasis most often takes place in the liver, where it is called colon metastasis in the liver. The second most-common location for colon metastasis is the lungs.

Minerals—*Nutrients,* such as iron, calcium and potassium; required by the body in small amounts.

N

Neoplasm—Any abnormal growth of new *tissue,* also called a *tumor.* A neoplasm may be *benign* or *malignant.* However, in current medical terminology, it is commonly used to refer to *cancer.*

Nutrient—The part of the food you eat that the body uses to grow, function and stay alive. The major classes of nutrients that the body needs are *proteins, carbohydrates, minerals, fats* and *vitamins.*

Nutrition—A three-part process that gives the body the *nutrients* it needs. First, you eat or drink food. Second, the body breaks the food down into nutrients. Third, the nutrients travel through the bloodstream to different parts of the body where they are used as "fuel." To give your body proper nutrition, you have to eat or drink enough of the foods that contain key nutrients.

O

Occult Blood Test (OCBT)—See *Fecal Occult Blood Test.*

Oncologist—Doctor who specializes in diagnosing and treating *cancer.*

P

Palliative Treatment, Palliative Therapy—*Treatments* used in advanced *cancer* situations to relieve pain and suffering rather than to cure. Palliative actions are undertaken to comfort the patient and to improve the quality of life. Examples include palliative *chemotherapy*, palliative *radiation* and palliative surgery.

Pathologist—Doctor who specializes in the analysis of body *tissue*. Tissue that is extracted from a patient is sent to a pathologist, who conducts a microscopic examination and determines whether it is *benign* or *malignant*. A pathology report is prepared to provide the patient's doctor with medical information to help determine the proper course of *treatment*. See also *Biopsy*.

Pedunculated Polyp—*Polyp* that resembles a mushroom. Grows on a stalk that connects the head of the polyp to the *bowel* wall. Illustration on page 22. See also *Adenoma; Hyperplastic Poly; Sessile Polyp*.

Physician Data Query (PDQ)—Computer data base used to store and retrieve information concerning detection, *diagnosis, treatment* and *prognosis* of *cancer*. Supported by the National Cancer Institute (NCI). Developed and updated with the assistance of more than 400 cancer specialists in the United States. Medical professionals can access the PDQ system through a computer located in an office, lab or home. Cancer patients and the general public can access PDQ information by calling the NCI's Cancer Information Service at 1-800-4-CANCER.

Polyp—Abnormal growth that protrudes from the inner lining of an organ such as the *colon*. Although the vast majority of newly discovered polyps are *benign*, there is always the possibility that benign polyps will become *malignant*. Scientists currently believe that most *cancers* of the *large bowel* evolve from *adenomatous* polyps. See also *Adenoma; Hyperplastic Polyp*.

Polypectomy—Procedure used to remove *polyps* during a *colonoscopy* or *sigmoidoscopy*. A wire loop is passed through the colonoscope or sigmoidoscope and a polyp is "lassoed" by placing the loop around the polyp. Using an electrical charge, the polyp is quickly and painlessly severed.

Potassium—A *mineral* the body needs for fluid balance and other essential functions.

Precursor—Something that precedes something else. For example, an *adenomatous polyp* is generally considered to be a precursor of cancer.

Procto (Procto exam, Proctosigmoidoscopy)—See *Sigmoidoscopy*.

Proctologist—Physician who specializes in diagnosing and treating problems of the *colon, rectum* and *anus*.

Prognosis—Prediction or medical statement explaining the likely outcome of disease or disorder in a particular patient.

Protein—One of the three *nutrients* that supply *calories* (energy) to the body. Protein is also an essential component of the body's *cells* and becomes a part of the muscle, bone, skin and blood. Approximately 12% to 15% of your total calories should come from protein. Excess protein will be stored as fat in the body, as will excess *fat* or *carbohydrate*. Primary sources of protein are meat, poultry, fish, milk, cheese, eggs, dried beans and peas. See also *Carbohydrate; Fat*.

Proximal Colon (Right Colon)—First part of the *large bowel*, consisting of the *cecum*, ascending colon and transverse colon. Illustration on page 9. See also *Distal Colon*.

R

Radiation Therapy (Cobalt Treatment, X-ray Therapy, Radiotherapy)— *Treatment* of *cancer* by using penetrating, high-energy rays or subatomic particles to control the disease. Radiation works by killing and eliminating cancer *cells* and *tumors*, shrinking tumors or preventing cancer cells from growing and dividing. Radiation can be used as a primary or *adjuvant* treatment. In treating *colorectal cancer*, radiation can be used before, during and after surgery. See also *External Radiation; Internal Radiation; Palliative Treatment*.

Radiologist—Physician with special training in analyzing diagnostic X-rays and performing specialized X-ray procedures.

Rectum—Organ in which solid food waste is stored until being excreted through the *anus*. See also *Digestive System; Large Bowel*.

Recurrence (Recurrent Cancer)—Reappearance of *cancer* after a period of time when there has been no evidence of cancer.

Remission—Partial shrinkage or complete disappearance of *cancer*, usually occurring as a result of *treatment*. Remission is a period when the disease is under control. Remission is not necessarily a cure. In general, five years without recurrence is considered a cure.

Resection—See *Bowel Resection*.

Right Colon—See *Proximal Colon*.

S

Screening—Search for disease in an apparently healthy person who has no *symptoms*. Screening can also refer to coordinated programs involving large populations where the objective is to detect disease in people who are not aware of its presence. The most common screening methods for *colorectal cancer* are the *digital rectal exam, fecal occult blood test* and *sigmoidoscopy*.

Secondary Cancer—See *Metastasis*.

Sessile Polyp—*Polyp* that is flat and grows directly on the wall of an organ such as the *large bowel*. Illustration on page 22. See also *Adenoma; Pedunculated Polyp; Hyperplastic Polyp*.

Sigmoidoscopy (Procto Exam, Procto, Proctosigmoidoscopy)—Exam in which a thin, lighted, *fiberoptic* tubular instrument called a *sigmoidoscope* is inserted into the *large bowel* through the *anus*. The doctor can look through the sigmoidoscope to perform a visual examination of the inner walls of the *rectum* and the lower portions of the *colon*. At maximum extension, the sigmoidoscope can investigate only about one-third the length of the large bowel. The older, limited, rigid sigmoidoscope should be avoided. The newer, safer, longer and more accurate flexible sigmoidoscope is recommended.

During a procto exam, the doctor can take a *biopsy* or remove a *polyp*, utilizing a procedure called *polypectomy*. It is generally recommended that anyone over the age of 50 should have a sigmoidoscopy every 3 to 5 years. See also *Colonoscopy*.

Small Bowel (Small Intestine)—Organ whose main function is to process food. Situated between the stomach and the *large bowel*, the small bowel is about 6 meters (20 feet) long. It is three to five times longer than the large bowel, but much smaller in circumference. By the time food travels through the small intestine, 90% to 95% of food has been processed. The *nutrients* and fluids have been extracted and sent to the bloodstream for distribution throughout the body. See also *Colon; Digestive System; Large Bowel*.

Sodium—A *mineral* required by the body to keep body fluids in balance; too much sodium can cause you to retain water. A diet with less salt may help some people reduce their risk of developing high blood pressure. Primary sources are salt; salted chips, crackers, pretzels and nuts; pickles and olives; some processed meats and cheeses; and many frozen meals and fast food.

Sphincter Muscle—Circular, clamp-like muscle that tightens and loosens around the *rectum*. Its purpose is to control excretion of waste.

Staging—Organized process of determining the extent *cancer* has spread. Staging involves many forms of medical investigation, including physical examinations, tests to measure liver or lung functions, blood tests, X-rays, *colonoscopies, biopsies*, scans and sometimes surgery. Takes into account how deeply the cancerous *tumor* has invaded the *bowel* wall and whether other organs or *lymph nodes* are involved. Defining the stage or phase of the spread of cancer helps determine the most appropriate *treatment* and the *prognosis*.

Dukes' *System* is a common staging method. It describes *colorectal-cancer* stages from Dukes' A through Dukes' D, with A being start-up cancer and D being the most serious cancer. The *TNM System* ranks the stages of cancer from 0 through IV, with 0 as the beginning phase of cancer.

Statistical Probability—Mathematically determined likelihood that some event will occur. For example, the statistical probability that someone living in the United States will get *colorectal cancer* is 5% to 6%.

Stoma—A surgically created opening in the abdomen that allows for removal of body wastes. See also *Colostomy*.

Stool—See *Feces*.

Stool-Blood Test—See *Fecal Occult Blood Test*.

Suture-Line cancer—Cancer which appears along the line where the bowel has been resewn following the removal of a cancerous section.

Symptom—Indication of a disease or disorder. For example, rectal bleeding is a symptom of *colorectal cancer*.

T

Tenesmus—Ineffectual and sometimes painful straining to excrete *feces*, coupled with a constant feeling of not being able to empty the *rectum* completely. *Symptom* of *colorectal cancer* and *polyps*.

Tissue—Group of similar *cells*.

TNM System—*Staging* system that describes how far *cancer* has spread in a patient. T refers to *tumor* size, N to *lymph node* involvement and M to *metastasis*. The TNM system defines cancer stages from Stage 0, beginning phase of cancer through Stage I, Stage II and Stage III to Stage IV, the most serious phase of cancer. See also *Dukes' System.*

Total Parenteral Nutrition (TPN)—Method of providing a patient all of the *nutrients* he or she needs through a needle in a vein. TPN may be used when the mouth, the stomach, or the bowel are sore from *cancer treatment.*

Treatment—Management and care of a patient. Combating of disease or disorder.

Tubular Cell Growth—The least-dangerous cell-growth pattern found in *colorectal cancer.* When viewed under a microscope, the *cells* appear tube-like in form. See also *Tubulovillous Cell Growth; Villous Cell Growth.*

Tubulovillous Cell Growth—One of three cell-growth patterns found in *colorectal polyps.* Comprised of a mixture of the patterns found in tubular and villous cell growth. See also *Tubular Cell Growth; Villous Cell Growth.*

Tumor—Term commonly used to describe *cancer.* However, the actual meaning of the term is "swelling" and it can be used to describe any lump or swelling regardless of whether it is *benign* or *malignant.* In other words, cancers could be called *tumors,* but not all tumors are cancer.

V

Villous Cell Growth—The most-dangerous cell-growth pattern found in *colorectal polyps.* When viewed under a microscope, the *cells* have a shaggy and frond-like appearance. See also *Tubular Cell Growth; Tubulovillous Cell Growth.*

Vitamins—Key *nutrients* that the body needs to grow and stay strong. The best source of vitamins, such as vitamins A, B, and C, is the foods we eat. Vitamin A occurs in two major forms: retinol, which is found in animal sources; and beta carotene, which is found in vegetable sources. This vitamin is important for normal mucous membranes, good vision, normal bone growth and healthy skin and hair. Primary sources for retinol are liver and fish-liver oils. Smaller amounts are also found in egg yolks, red meats, butter and margarine. Primary sources for beta carotene are carrots, broccoli, deep-green and leafy vegetables, cantaloupe and apricots.

The B vitamins include thiamine, riboflavin and niacin. They are all important in the processing of nutrients and the maintenance of healthy blood vessels and *cells,* teeth and gums, and healthy nervous and cardiovascular systems. Primary sources are whole grains, eggs, vegetables, fish and poultry.

Vitamin C is also known as *ascorbic acid.* It is essential for maintaining healthy teeth, gums and bones; for building strong cells and blood vessels; for healing wounds and broken bones; and for resisting *infections.* Primary sources are citrus fruits, strawberries, broccoli and tomatoes.

W

Wedge Resection—Surgical removal of a *tumor* and surrounding mass of *tissue.* Sometimes used as a *treatment* for beginning *stages* of *colorectal cancer.*

Bibliography

(Only the first author of each work is provided.)

ARTICLES, PAMPHLETS, REPORTS

Achkar, E. "Colonoscopy—Who Can Avoid It?" *Gastroenterology*, June 1989, 1613-1619.

Allen-Mersh, T. "Colorectal Cancer—Diagnosis, Management, and Prognosis." *Comprehensive Therapy*, Jan 1991, 3-7.

American Cancer Society. *Adjuvant Treatment*. Publication #5011, 1993.
    Cancer Facts And Figures—1994.
    Cancer Facts And Figures—1995.
    Cancer Related Check-Ups. Publication #2070-CE, 1980.
    Colorectal Cancer: Diagnosis. Publication #409576, Aug 1993.
    Colorectal Cancer: Prognosis. Publication #409578, Apr 27, 1992.
    Colorectal Cancer: Staging. Publication #409568, Sep 1993.
    Colorectal Cancer: Treatment. Publication #409577, Aug 1993.
    Colostomy—A Guide. Publication #4703, Feb 1991.
    Eating Smart. Publication #2042-LE, 1987.
    Facts On Colorectal Cancer. Publication #2004-LE, 1993.
    Nutrition, Common Sense And Cancer. Publication #2096-LE, 1984.
    Talking With Your Doctor. Publication #4638, 1994.

American Society of Colon and Rectal Surgeons. *Questions and Answers—Colorectal Cancer.*

American Society of Colon and Rectal Surgeons. *Your Doctor is a Colon and Rectal Surgeon*, 1990.

Angier, N. "Scientists Isolate Gene That Causes Cancer of Colon." *The New York Times*, Dec 3, 1993, 1.

Asburn, H. "Management of Recurrent and Metastatic Colorectal Carcinoma." *Surgical Clinics of North America*, Feb. 1993, 143-165.

Atkin, W. "Prevention of Colorectal Cancer By Once Only Sigmoidoscopy." *The Lancet*, Mar 20, 1993, 736-742.

Atkin, W. "Long-Term Risk Of Colorectal Cancer After Excision Of Rectosigmoid Adenomas." *The New England Journal Of Medicine*, Mar 1992, 658-662.

"Bowel Cancer: Nipping It In The Bud." *Harvard Medical School Health Letter*, Sep 1989.

Brady, A. "Colorectal Cancer Overlooked at Barium Enema Examination and Colonoscopy; A Continuing Perceptual Problem." *Radiology*, Aug 1984, 374-378.

Brenner, D. "Colon Cancer." *Coping*, July/Aug 1994, 60.

Brint, S. "Colorectal Cancer Screening: Is One-Year Surveillance Sigmoidoscopy Necessary." *The American Journal of Gastroenterology*, Aug 3, 1993, 2019-2020.

Brody, J. "Report Calls Simple Test Effective for Reducing Colon Cancer Deaths." *The New York Times*, May 13, 1993, 1

Brody, J. "Screening for Cancer of the Colon: Range of Options." *The New York Times*, Mar 10, 1993, B7.

Burris, J. "Mass Colorectal Cancer Screening: Choosing an Effective Strategy." *AAOHN Journal*, Apr 1993, 186-191.

"Cancer Team Targets Colorectal Gene." *Science News*, Mar 1994, 121.

Cauffman, J. "Screening Asymptomatic Patients for Colorectal Lesions." *Family Practice Research Journal*, Mar 1994, 77-79.

Carey, A. "Colonoscopy—Who Can Avoid It?" (Letter) *Gastroenterology*, June 1989, 1613-1614.

Chen, F. "Colonoscopic Follow-Up of Colorectal Carcinoma." *Diseases of the Colon & Rectum*, Jan 1994, 568-574.

Chu, K. "Temporal Patterns in Colorectal Cancer Incidence, Survival and Mortality." *Journal of the National Cancer Institute,* July 6, 1994, 997-1003.

Clayman, C. "Mass Screening for Colorectal Cancer: Are We Ready?" *Journal of the American Medical Association*, Jan 27, 1989, 609.

"Clues To Colon Cancer." *Nutrition Action Healthletter*, Mar 1990, 5.

Cohen, A. "Rectal Cancer: Quality Considerations in Surgical Therapy." *News From The Commission on Cancer*. American College of Surgeons, 1994.

"The Colon Book." *Krames Communications*, 1991.

"Colon Cancer: Molecular Analysis Marches On." *The Lancet,* June 3, 1989, 1236.

"Colonic Polyps, Occult Blood And Cancer." *JAMA*, Jan 27, 1989, 76-84.

"Colonoscopy." *Krames Communications*, 1990.

"Colonoscopy In Asymptomatic Patients." *Patient Care*, Apr 30, 1991, 23-24.

"Colorectal Cancer Comes of Age." *The New England Journal of Medicine*, May 13, 1993, 1416.

"Colorectal Cancer: New Evidence For The Adenoma/Carcinoma Sequence." *The Lancet,* July 25, 1992, 210-211.

"Could Aspirin Really Prevent Colon Cancer." *The New England Journal Of Medicine*, Dec 5, 1991, 1644-1645.

Cummings, B. "Radiation Therapy for Colorectal Cancer." *Surgical Clinics Of North America*, Feb 1993, 167-179.

Cummings, J. "Colon Cancer Risk And Dietary Intake of Nonstarch Polysaccharides (Dietary Fiber)." *Gastroenterology*, Oct 1992, 1782-1789.

Curless, R. "Colorectal Carcinoma; Elderly Patients." *Age and Ageing*, Mar 1994, 102-104.

De Cosse, J. "Colorectal Cancer: Detection, Treatment, and Rehabilitation." *A Cancer Journal For Clinicians*, Jan/Feb 1994, 27-37.

Desforges, J. "Screening For Colorectal Cancer." *The New England Journal Of Medicine*, July 1991, 37-41.

"Diverticulosis And Diverticulitis." *Krames Communications*, 1993.

Eckhausser, M. "Laser Therapy Of Colorectal Carcinomas." *Surgical Clinics Of North America*, Jan 1992, 597-606.

Eddy, D. "Screening Cancer in a High Risk Population." *Gastroenterology*, Nov 1987, 682-687.

Enker, W. "Bowel Function And Dietary Fiber." Paper given to author.

Evans, J. "Management And Survival Of Carcinoma Of The Colon." *Annals Of Surgery*, Dec 1978, 716-720.

Ferguson, E. "Preventing Colorectal Cancer." *Southern Medical Journal*, Nov 1990, 1295-1298.

Ferrucci, J. "Screening for Colorectal Cancer." *Radiologic Clinics of North America*, Nov 1993, 1189-1195.

Fleischer, D. "Detection And Surveillance Of Colorectal Cancer." *JAMA*, Jan 27, 1989, 580-585.

Fong, Y. "Surgical Treatment of Colorectal Metastases to the Liver." *A Cancer Journal for Clinicians*, Jan/Feb 1995, 50-56.

Forman, W. "The Role of Chemotherapy and Adjuvant Therapy in the Management of Colorectal Cancer." *Cancer Supplement,* Oct 1, 1994, 2151-2153.

Friend, T. "Tenacious Gene Team Behind Colon Cancer Breakthrough." *USA Today*, Dec 14, 1993, 5.

Gambone, J. "A Consumer's Guide to Better Medical Decisions." *Great Performances, Inc.*, 1993.

Gareural, H. "Aspirin in the Prevention of Colorectal Cancer." *Annals of Internal Medicine*, Aug 15, 1994, 303-309.

Giovannucci, E. "Aspirin Use and the Risk for Colorectal Cancer and Adenoma in Male Health Professionals." *Annals of Internal Medicine*, Aug 15, 1994, 241-245.

Giovannucci, E. "Relationship of Diet To Risk of Colorectal Adenoma In Men." *JAMA*, Mar 25, 1992, 1595.

Greenberg, E. "Prospects for Preventing Colorectal Cancer Death." *Journal of the National Cancer Institute*, Aug 4, 1993, 1182-1184.

Gschvantler, M. "Detection of Colorectal Adenomas By Fecal Occult Blood Tests." (Letter) *Gastroenterology*, Jan. 1994, 279-286.

"The Hemorrhoid Book." *Krames Communications*, 1991.

Ho, R. "The Future Direction of Clinical Trials." *Cancer*, Nov 1, 1994, 2734-2748.

Jenks, S. "After Early Hype, Interferons Spark Interest." *Journal of the National Cancer Institute*, May 19, 1993, 773-775.

Kaps, E. "The Role of the Support Group—Us Too." *Cancer Supplement,* Oct 1 1994, 2188-2189.

Kewenter, J. "Follow-Up After Screening For Colorectal Neoplasms with Fecal Occult Blood Testing In a Controlled Trial." *Diseases of the Colon and Rectum*, Feb 1994, 115-118.

Knight, K. "Occult Blood Screening for Colorectal Cancer." *JAMA*, Jan 27, 1989, 586-590.

Kolata, G. "Cancer Causing Gene Found, With A Clue To How It Works." *The New York Times*, May 6, 1993, 1.

Kronborg, O. "Optimal Follow-Up in Colorectal Cancer Patients." *Seminars in Surgical Oncology*, May/June 1994, 217-224.

Lang, C. "Fecal Occult Blood Screening for Colorectal Cancer." *JAMA*, Apr 6, 1994, 1011-1016.

Levin, B. "Colorectal Cancer Screening." *Cancer*, Aug 1, 1993, 1056-1060.

Levin, B. "Nutrition and Colorectal Cancer." *Cancer Supplement*, Sep 15, 1992, 1723-1726.

Levin, B. "Screening Sigmoidoscopy for Colorectal Cancer." *The New England Journal of Medicine*, Mar 5, 1992, 700-701.

Lieberman, D. "Screening/Early Detection Model for Colorectal Cancer." *Cancer Supplement*, Oct 1, 1994, 2023-2026.

"Lower GI Endoscopy." *Krames Communications*, 1983.

MacCarty, M. "Colorectal Cancer: The Case for Barium Enema." *Mayo Clinic Proceedings*, Mar 1992, 253-257.

Mandel, J. "Reducing Mortality From Colorectal Cancer by Screening for Fecal Occult Blood." *The New England Journal of Medicine*, May 13, 1993, 1365-1371.

Mandel, J. "Screening for Colorectal Cancer: Which Test is Best?" (Letter) *JAMA*, Oct 12, 1994, 1099.

Maule, W. "Screening for Colorectal Cancer by Nurse Endoscopists." *The New England Journal Of Medicine*, Jan 20, 1994, 183-186.

Meagher, A. "Does Colonoscopic Polypectomy Reduce the Incidence of Colorectal Carcinoma." *Australian and New Zealand Journal of Surgery*, June 1994, 400-404.

Milene, D. "Right, Left, Right or Wrong; Debate Whirls Around Colorectal Cancer Distribution." *Journal of the National Cancer Institute*, Oct 5, 1994, 1442-1443.

Moran, J. "Utilization of Sigmoidoscopy." (Letter) *Canadian Medical Association Journal*, May 15, 1994, 1544.

Myers, R. "Adherence to Continuous Screening For Colorectal Neoplasia." *Medical Care*, Jan 1993, 508-510.

Nathanson, S. "Is There a Role for Clinical Prognostic Factors in Staging Patients With Colorectal Cancer." *Seminars in Surgical Oncology*, May/June 1994, 176-182.

National Cancer Institute. *Cancer Facts.* July 26, 1994.

Cancer Facts—Biological Therapies: Newest Form of Cancer Treatment. Reference #7.2, 1988.

Cancer of the Colon and Rectum. Publication #92-95, Oct 1991.

Colon Cancer. PDQ, Aug 1993.

Colon Cancer Prognosis. PDQ, Aug 1994.

"Colonoscopies and Polyp Removal Help Prevent Cancer." *To Your Health ... News from the Polyp Prevention Trial.* 1994.

Colorectal Cancer: Treatment Overview. Publication #409577, Oct 1993.

Diagnosis, Colon Cancer. PDQ, Aug 1994.

Diagnosis, Rectal Cancer. PDQ, Dec 1994.

Diet and Large-Bowel Cancer—The Facts Behind the PPT, 1994.

Eating Hints, Recipes & Tips for Better Nutrition During Cancer Treatment.
   Publication #92-2079, 1990.
Good Fiber-a-tions. Polyp Prevention Trial, 1994.
Radiation Therapy and You. Publication #94-2227, 1993.
Rectal Cancer Prognosis. PDQ, Aug 1994.
What Are Clinical Trials All About? Publication #92-2706, June 1992.
What You Need to Know About Cancer of the Colon and Rectum. Publication
   #90-1552, Nov 1989.
Nelson, R. "Diet and Adenomatous Polyps Risk." *Seminars in Surgical Oncology*,
   May/June 1994, 165-175.
O'Brien, M. "The National Polyp Study." *Gastroenterology*, Nov 1990, 371-377.
Ott, J. "Role of the Barium Enema in Colorectal Carcinoma." *Radiologic Clinics of
   North America*, Nov 1993, 1293-1307.
Paganni-Hill, A. "Aspirin and the Prevention of Colorectal Cancer: A Review of
   the Evidence." *Seminars in Surgical Oncology*, May/June 1994, 158-163.
"Positive For Occult Blood: What Next?" *Patient Care*, Dec 15, 1991, 167-168.
Ranschoff, D. "The Case for Colorectal Cancer Screening." *Hospital Practice
   (Office Edition)*, Aug 15, 1994, 25-28.
Ranschoff, D. "Screening for Colorectal Cancer." *The New England Journal of
   Medicine*, July 4, 1991, 37-41.
Ranschoff, D. "Small Adenomas Detected During Fecal Occult Blood Test
   Screening For Colorectal Cancer." *JAMA*, July 4, 1990, 76-78.
Rex, D. "Endoscopic Screening for Colorectal Cancer." *Indiana Medicine*, Jan/Feb
   1994, 68-73.
Rex, D. "Screening Colonoscopy In Asymptomatic Average-Risk Persons With
   Negative Fecal Occult Blood Tests." *Gastroenterology*, Aug 1991, 64-67.
Reynolds, T. "Evidence Emerges: Colorectal Cancer Screening Reduces Death."
   Journal of the National Cancer Institute, May 19, 1993, 770-772.
Ruddy, B. "Effect of Dietary Fiber on Colonic Bacterial Enzymes and Bile Acids
   in Reaction to Colon Cancer." *Gastroenterology*, Mar 1992, 1475-1480.
Sagamoto, M. "Screening Flexible Sigmoidoscopy in a Low-Risk, Highly
   Screened Population." *Journal of Family Practice*, Mar 1994, 245.
Sandler, R. "Diet and Risk of Colorectal Adenomas: Macronutrients, Cholesterol
   and Fiber." *Journal of the National Cancer Institute*, June 2, 1993, 884-890.
Schrock, T. "Colonoscopy for Colorectal Cancer: Too Much, Too Little, Just
   Right." *Gastrointestinal Endoscopy*, Nov 6, 1993, 848-850.
"Screening For Bowel Cancer." *Harvard Medical School Health Letter,* Apr 1986.
Selby, J. "A Case-Control Study of Screening Sigmoidoscopy and Mortality from
   Colorectal Cancer." *The New England Journal of Medicine*, Mar 5, 1992, 653-537.
Selby, J. "Effect of Fecal Occult Blood Testing on Mortality From Colorectal
   Cancer." *Annals of Internal Medicine*, Jan 1993, 1-5.
Selby, J. "Sigmoidoscopy In The Periodic Health Examination of Asymptomatic
   Adults." *JAMA*, Jan 27, 1989, 595-601.
Sexe, R. "Rectal Cancer." *Postgraduate Medicine*, July 1993, 189-191.

Shimbo, T. "Cost-Effectiveness Analysis of Strategies for Colorectal Cancer Screening in Japan." *International Journal of Technology in Health Care,* Oct 3, 1994, 359-375.

Simon, J. "Colonic Polyps, Occult Blood, and Chance." *JAMA,* July 4, 1990, 84-85.

"Simple Cancer Test That Saves Lives." *The John Hopkins Medical Letter,* Sep 1992, 3.

Smigel, K. "Group Defines Directions for Colorectal Cancer Screening." *Journal of the National Cancer Institute,* July 6, 1994, 958-960.

Snider, M. "Colorectal Cancer May Have Link To Smoking." *USA Today,* Feb 2, 1994, 1.

Solomon, M. "Periodic Health Examination, 1994 Update: 2 Screening Strategies for Colorectal Cancer." *Canadian Medical Association Journal,* June 15, 1994, 1961-1969.

St. John, J. "Cancer Risk In Relatives Of Patients with Common Colorectal Cancer." *Annals Of Internal Medicine,* May 15, 1993, 785.

Steele, G. "Standard Postoperative Monitoring of Patients After Primary Resection of Colon and Rectum Cancer." *Cancer Supplement,* June 15, 1993, 4225-4235.

Steele, G. "The National Cancer Data Base on Colorectal Cancer." *Cancer,* Oct 1, 1994, 1979-1989.

Stroehlein, J. "Hemoccult Stool Test's False Negative Results Due to Storage of Specimens." *Mayo Clinic Proceedings,* May 1975.

"Test After Colon Surgery is Ineffective, Study Says." *The New York Times,* Aug 25, 1993, B7.

Threhu, E. "Cost of Screening for Colorectal Cancer." *Southern Medical Journal,* Mar 1992, 248-253.

Tierney, R. "The Adenoma to Carcinoma Sequence." *Surgery, Gynecology, and Obstetrics,* July 1990, 81-91.

Trock, B. "Dietary Fiber, Vegetables and Colon Cancer: Critical Review And Meta-Analyses Of The Epidemiologic Evidence." *Journal Of The National Cancer Institute,* Apr 18, 1990, 650-657.

Turk, P. "Results of Surgical Treatment of Nonhepatic Recurrence of Colorectal Cancer." *Cancer Supplement,* Jan 15, 1993, 426-427.

Vaughn, D. "Nonsurgical Management Of Recurrent Colorectal Cancer." *Nonsurgical Management, Cancer Supplement,* June 15, 1993, 4278.

Vernova, A. "Current Follow-up Strategies After Resection Of Colon Cancer." *Diseases Of The Colon And Rectum,* June 1994, 578-583.

Wherry, D. "The Yield of Flexible Fiberoptic Sigmoidoscopy In The Detection of Asymptomatic Colorectal Neoplasia." *Surgical Endoscopy,* May 1994, 393-396.

White, L. "Cancer Risk and Early Detection Assessment." *Seminars in Oncology Nursing,* Aug 1993, 188-191.

Whynes, D. "Cost Savings in Mass Population Screening for Colorectal Cancer Resulting from the Early Detection and Excision of Adenomas." *Health Economics,* Apr 1992, 53-61.

Winawer, S. "Colorectal Cancer Comes of Age." *The New England Journal of Medicine*, May 13, 1993, 1416-1417.

Winawer, S. "Prevention of Colorectal Cancer by Colonoscopic Polypectomy." *The New England Journal of Medicine,* Dec 30, 1993, 1977-1981.

Witt, M. "Current Management of Adults With Colorectal Cancer." *Nursing,* Apr 1993, 105-108.

Wood, A. "Chemotherapy for Colorectal Cancer." *The New England Journal Of Medicine*, Apr 21, 1994, 1136.

BOOKS

Altman, R. *The Cancer Dictionary*. New York: Facts on File, 1992

American Cancer Society. *The Cancer Book*. New York: Doubleday, 1986.

Bair, F. *Cancer Source Book*. Detroit: Omnigraphics, 1990.

Balch, J. *Prescriptions for Nutritional Healing*. Garden City Park, NY: Avery Publishing Group, 1993.

Becker, G. *Antioxidant Pocket Counter*. New York: Times Books, 1993.

Belcher, Ann. *Cancer Nursing*. New York: Mosby Year Book, 1992.

Bellerson, K. *The Complete & Up-To-Date Fat Book*. Garden City Park, NY: Avery Publishing Group, 1991.

Brody, J. *Nutrition Book*. New York: Bantam Books, 1991.

Carper, J. *Total Nutrition Guide*. New York: Bantam Books, 1987.

Clyne, R. *Coping With Cancer: Making Sense Of It All*. San Francisco: Thorsons Publishing, 1986.

Cohen, A. *Cancer Of The Colon, Rectum & Anus*. New York: McGraw-Hill, 1994.

Complete Book Of Cancer Prevention. Emmaus, PA: Rodale Press, 1988.

DeCosse, J. *Cancer Book*. New York: Doubleday, 1986.

DeVita, V., Jr. *Cancer: Principles And Practice Of Oncology*. Philadelphia: J.B. Lippincott Company, 1993.

Dollinger, M. *Everyone's Guide To Cancer Therapy*. Toronto: Andrews & McMeed, 1991.

Dreher, H. *Your Defense Against Cancer*. New York: Harper Collins, 1994.

Faivre, J. *Causation & Prevention Of Colorectal Cancer*. New York: Elsevier Science, 1987.

Fat And Cholesterol Counter. New York: Times Books, 1991.

Friedberg, G. *Cancer Answers*. New York: W.H. Freeman & Company, 1992.

Garrison, R. *The Nutrition Desk Reference*. New Canaan, CT: Keats Pub., 1985.

Haas, E. *Staying Healthy With Nutrition*. New York: Times Books, 1990.

Handler, S. *The Doctor's Vitamin and Mineral Encyclopedia*. New York: Simon & Schuster, 1990.

Hardcastle, J. *Colorectal Cancer: Textbook For General Practitioners*. New York: Springer-Verlag, 1993.

Harplam, W. *Diagnosis Cancer*. New York: W.W. Norton & Company, 1992.

Harwell, A. *When Your Friend Gets Cancer: How You Can Help.* Wheaton, IL: Harold Shaw Publishers, 1989.

Johnson, J. *Staying Healthy with Cancer.* Minnetonka, MN: Chronimed Publishing, 1994.

Kamen, B. *New Facts About Fiber: Health Builder, Disease Fighter, Vital Nutrient.* Novato, CA: Nutrition Encounter, 1991.

Kaufman, D. *Surviving Cancer.* Washington, DC: Acropolis Books, 1989.

Lazlo, J. *Understanding Cancer.* New York: Harper & Row, 1987.

Le Shan, L. *Cancer At A Turning Point: A Handbook For People With Cancer, Their Families,* And Health Professionals. New York: Dutton, 1989.

Mandell. *Vitamin Bible.* New York: Warner Books, 1991.

McAllister, R. *Cancer.* New York: Basic Books, 1993.

Menko, F. *Genetics of Colorectal Cancer for Clinical Practice.* Notre Dame, IN: Kluwer Academic Publishers, 1990.

Mora, M. *Choices, Realistic Alternatives.* New York: Avon Books, 1991.

Mosby Medical Encyclopedia, The. New York: Plume Books, 1992.

Moss, R. *Cancer Therapy.* Brooklyn: Equinox Press, 1992.

Natrow, A. *The Fat Attack Plan.* New York: Pocket Books, 1990.

Pelton, R. *Alternatives to Cancer Therapy: The Complete Guide To Non-Traditional Treatments.* New York: Simon & Schuster, 1994.

Podell, S. *Fat Counter.* New York: Doubleday, 1992.

Rosenbaum, E. *A Comprehensive Guide For Cancer Patients And Their Families.* Menlo Park, CA: Bull Publishing Company, 1980.

Sattilaro, A. *Living Well Naturally.* New York: Houghton Mifflin Company, 1984.

Sheel, R. *Handbook of Cancer Chemotherapy.* New York: Little, Brown and Company, 1991.

Sheldon, S. *The Diagnosis Is Cancer:* A Psychological And Legal Resource Handbook for Cancer Patients. Menlo Park, CA: Bull Publishing Company, 1986.

Siegel, M. *The Cancer Patient's Handbook.* New York: Walker and Company, 1986.

Simone, C. *Cancer & Nutrition.* Garden City Park, NY: Avery Publishing Group, 1992.

Simonton, C. *The Healing Journey.* New York: Bantam Books, 1992.

Stedman's Medical Dictionary. Baltimore: William Wood and Company, 1990.

Watkin, D. *Handbook of Nutrition and Aging.* Park Ridge, NJ: Noyes Publishers, 1983.

Webster's Medical Desk Dictionary. Springfield, MA: Merriam-Webster Inc., 1986.

Weil, A. *Natural Health, Natural Medicine.* New York: Houghton Mifflin Company, 1990.

INDEX